BUMPS &
BURPEES

BUMPS & BURPEES

Your guide to staying strong, fit and
happy throughout pregnancy

CHARLIE
BARKER

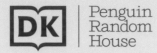

Penguin
Random
House

Senior Acquisitions Editor Stephanie Milner
Managing Art Editor Bess Daly
Project Designer Karen Constanti
Project Editor Dawn Bates
Jacket Designer and illustrator Amy Cox
Jackets Coordinator Lucy Philpott
Senior Production Editor Tony Phipps
Production Controller Rebecca Parton
Art Director Maxine Pedliham
Publishing Director Katie Cowan

Photography by Claire Pepper,
except page 216 by Agata Sroka
Make-up by Bianca Mitchell

First published in Great Britain in 2021 by
Dorling Kindersley Limited
DK, One Embassy Gardens, 8 Viaduct Gardens,
London, SW11 7BW

The authorised representative in the EEA is
Dorling Kindersley Verlag GmbH. Arnulfstr. 124,
80636 Munich, Germany

A CIP catalogue record for this book
is available from the British Library.
ISBN: 978-0-2414-9111-9

Printed and bound in China
For the curious
www.dk.com

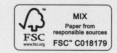

This book was made with Forest
Stewardship Council ™ certified
paper – one small step in DK's
commitment to a sustainable future.
For more information go to
www.dk.com/our-green-pledge

Disclaimer: The information in this book has been compiled as general guidance on the specific
subjects addressed. Neither the publisher nor the author is engaged in providing specific
professional advice to individual readers. The ideas, advice, and suggestions contained in this book
are not intended as a substitute for consulting with your doctor. Please consult your healthcare
provider before undertaking any of the exercises, techniques, and alternative therapies set out in
this book, and consult your GP before changing, stopping, or starting any medical treatment. So far
as the author is aware, the information given is correct and up to date as at February 2021. The
author and publisher disclaim, as far as the law allows, any liability for any loss or damage allegedly
arising from the use or misuse of any information or suggestion contained in this book.

CONTENTS

INTRODUCTION

Hello! If you're reading this book, then most likely congratulations are in order. If you're not pregnant yet, but preparing yourself ahead of time, that's great!

First, let me tell you a bit about me… I'm a personal trainer who specializes in pre- and postnatal fitness and the founder of Bumps & Burpees. As well as helping women to exercise safely and stay fit and strong throughout pregnancy and after the birth, my main aim is to encourage and empower pregnant women to feel strong on the inside as well as the outside at a time when so much is changing and feels out of their control.

Although the main focus of this book is pre- and post-natal fitness, I also share with you my experience of going through pregnancy – the ups, the downs, and the quite frankly strange things that happen to our bodies and minds in those life-changing months. I know that it is not all about feeling glowing and amazing, and that some days are really tough.

No matter what your circumstances, it is completely normal to feel so many different emotions during pregnancy – excitement and joy, but also anxiety and uncertainty. It can also feel difficult and frustrating if you're trying to keep your pregnancy a secret until your first scan. It may be that you aren't overcome with happiness, even if it is something you have longed for your whole life, and that can feel really confusing. Be reassured that it is normal for emotions to come and go and that is okay. As they do, I want you to feel supported by this book and part of a community of women who understand what you are going through.

I had a bit of a rocky journey to pregnancy and it was during this time

IT IS COMPLETELY NORMAL TO FEEL SO MANY DIFFERENT EMOTIONS DURING PREGNANCY.

that I realized how much support I needed. I often found it easier to seek advice from those that weren't closest to me. I took to social media and was welcomed into the most wonderful community of new and expectant mothers, many whom had been through a similar journey to me. It felt like they held my hand through it all and this is what I want this book to be for you too. I want you to know that I am right here with you on this crazy rollercoaster!

HOW TO USE THIS BOOK

This book it is not a 'how to' because there is no one way to do pregnancy – it is simply a guide to help you. The information is organized by trimester and at the start of each one you will find an idea of what to expect in the coming months. I share my experience of pregnancy, before giving you guidance on exercise for that trimester and a selection of workouts to choose from. There are 12 workouts in each trimester, but there is no pressure to complete them all. For how to do each exercise, see the Pose Directory on pages 36–61.

If you're coming to this book later in pregnancy, it is important to start in the correct trimester to ensure that the workouts are right for you and your bump

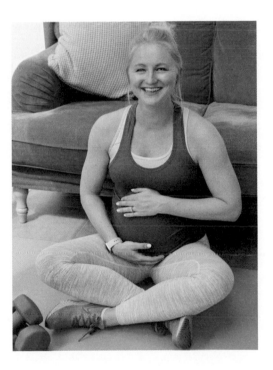

at that stage. If you are feeling rotten or exhausted, listen to your body and rest. I didn't stick to a rigid exercise routine during pregnancy – some weeks I felt great so I did more and others I did a minimal amount. Some days you may want to just do gentle stretching – see the Warm Up and Cool Down exercises on pages 26–33. You will need a small looped resistance band and dumbbells for some exercises – the size will be dependent on your strength. If you are a beginner, start with the lowest dumbbell weight and increase it when you can. To take it easier, use one weight. Familiarize yourself with the safety guidelines below before doing the workouts.

EXERCISING SAFELY

Many women ask if it is safe to exercise during pregnancy and the short answer is "Yes", unless it is against medical advice. In fact, the benefits outweigh the risks, which is why the UK government's Chief Medical Officer recommends 150 minutes of moderate intensity activity per week throughout pregnancy. There are a huge number of benefits to staying active:

- Improved cardiovascular fitness, which will help you carry around the extra weight of the baby, and prepare you for the physical exertion of labour and birth.
- Improved muscular strength to support your body as your bump grows and your posture changes, as well as preparing

you for lugging around car seats and buggies in the months to come.
- A lowered risk of developing gestational diabetes.
- Helps to prevent or alleviate symptoms of prenatal depression – those endorphins are so needed some days.

Moderate intensity is open to interpretation and the extent to which you can exercise will depend on how fit and used to exercising you are already. As a general guideline, aim to work to 70 per cent capacity – never push yourself to 100 per cent. Throughout a workout, tune into and listen to your body. Remember, pain is there to tell you something, so don't push through it. If a certain exercise causes you discomfort, try to adapt it or leave it out altogether for now. Your body will tell you if something doesn't feel right – it is just about listening to it.

Always stay hydrated before, during, and after exercising, and adequately fuel yourself. Whether you eat before or after will depend on what works best for you. Some women find that without eating first, they feel quite nauseous.

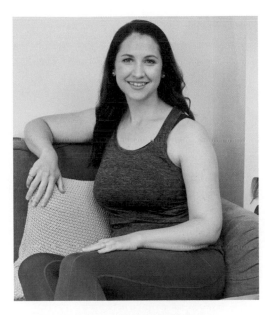

EXPERT **ADVICE**

I have been working alongside Clare Bourne, a pelvic health physiotherapist, for a long time and am thrilled that throughout this book you will benefit from her advice too. As well as working with pre- and postnatal women for years, Clare is the mother of two little ones herself so brings her personal experience. A pelvic health physiotherapist can treat a range of conditions that can cause pain and discomfort during pregnancy, and help if you are having difficulty with those all-important pelvic floor exercises.

ACTIVITIES TO AVOID

- Workouts where you are going to seriously overheat – only exercise in a very hot climate if you are used to it.
- Activities with a high risk of falling, such as horse-riding and gymnastics.
- Contact sports, where there is a risk of your bump being hit.
- Sky-diving and scuba-diving.
- Exercising at a very high altitude, unless you are acclimatized to it.

- After 16 weeks, exercises that involve lying on your back for longer than a few minutes. This causes the weight of the bump to press on the main blood vessel bringing blood back to your heart. It can cause low blood pressure and dizziness. I have adapted the workouts to take this into account.

MY ROCKY
PREGNANCY JOURNEY

I had dreamt of being a mum for as long as I could remember. I spent my teenage years babysitting and loved getting involved. Nothing phased me – I could handle teething babies, toddler tantrums, and even nappy explosions! I am the oldest of four siblings and always pictured myself having a big family of my own one day. When I began working with expectant and new mums, straight away I knew I loved helping them through this amazingly emotional time in their lives. I was very aware of the struggles some of the women had gone through to have their babies, but never imagined it would also happen to me. You just don't, do you?

PLANNING A FAMILY

I met my lovely husband George on the first day of university, and 10 years later we were married and keen to start a family right away. Little did we know that we were about to enter the most trying and emotional time of our lives. We fell pregnant the first month we tried. I couldn't believe it and was actually a little stunned by how easy it was, as I knew that this isn't always the case. We were over the moon, but decided to keep it to ourselves for a few weeks. Sadly, we didn't even get to that point as I started to bleed just over a week later. My doctor confirmed I was most likely

IT MADE US BOTH
REALIZE THAT BEING PARENTS
WAS THE ONE THING
WE WANTED AND
WE WERE READY.

having a miscarriage and advised me to wait it out at home, unless the pain became unbearable. I felt such overwhelming sadness, but it was accompanied with an understanding of how common this was and that we just had to try again. It made us both realize that being parents was the one thing we wanted and we were ready.

The very next month I found out that I was pregnant again. This time the excitement was accompanied with anxiety, for us both. Each day that I didn't bleed felt like a triumph in those first few weeks, and there wasn't one toilet trip when I didn't hold my breath dreading the worst.

As time went by, all the textbook pregnancy symptoms started and this is when I began to allow the hope back in and get more excited. It wasn't until a scan at 11 weeks that we were told that we had miscarried again, but my body had missed it. The baby was still in my tummy, but no longer alive. I say 'we' on purpose here because for so long I would say "I miscarried" and place all the blame on myself, and it changed everything for me when I started to say "we" and we began to go through things together as a team. What came next was probably the worst thing we have ever been through emotionally and it's something many women have spoken to me about since. We are all in agreement that no woman should ever have to give birth to a still-born child, no matter how far along they are. It is something I can never unsee, and will never forget. It took a long time for George and I to come to terms with

that and we decided to give trying for a baby a break. Part of me just wanted to try again straight away, but I knew I wasn't mentally strong enough for the emotions that come with it, so we agreed to take some time to just be us again. This was our best decision. We took a few months to get back to ourselves – we saw family, drank Pimms with friends, went on holiday. It wasn't all plain sailing though – those emotions didn't just vanish – but over time they became much less prevalent in our everyday lives. Eventually we felt ready to try again.

MORE HEARTACHE

We didn't seem to have too much of a problem getting pregnant – it happened very quickly again. Seeing those two lines on a pregnancy test filled us with joy, but I immediately felt the panic set in and I found myself doing as little as I physically could, hoping that this would help the baby stay in there. It didn't. Little over a week later, just before doing a talk about pregnancy to hundreds of women with bumps, I started

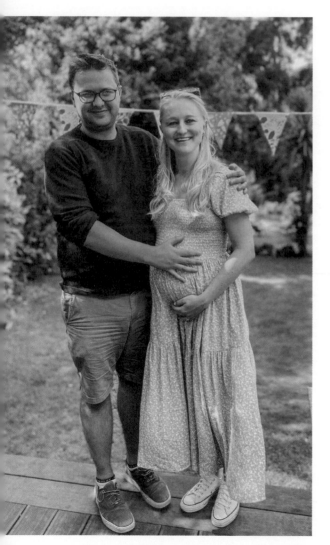

to bleed again. It was like a bad dream. I couldn't believe it; my heart sank having to tell George and then watch his heart sink too. We did a pregnancy test to double-check and it was just torture seeing it say "not pregnant" and realize that we were in this position again. This miscarriage wasn't as traumatic physically and was over pretty quickly, but it was the first time I thought to myself, "Will we ever be able to have a baby?" It was also the first time I doubted my body, which felt awful. I cried and cried for a week or two afterwards. I saw pregnant women everywhere – on social media, when I was walking down the street – it seemed like the whole world was pregnant.

SPECIALIST HELP

When all the NHS testing came back clear and showed no issues, I decided to take matters into my own hands. We were told to keep on trying, but I just felt like something was up. My gut was telling me that I would keep on miscarrying and I couldn't bear to put us through any more heartache. My good friend and

A FEW WEEKS LATER A SCAN SHOWED A LITTLE HEART BEATING AWAY AND WE COULD HAVE SCREAMED FROM THE ROOFTOPS. I WAS IN TOTAL DISBELIEF.

acupuncturist recommended a doctor who had a great track record in helping couples who suffered with recurrent miscarriage. I researched him for days and days before finally making an appointment. He was very popular, so we couldn't see him for eight weeks, and little did I know I would be pregnant again by that time.

The doctor ran some tests and found out that my immune system seemed to be attacking each pregnancy with a high number of natural killer cells, so we supported that with a concoction of steroids and intralipid drips, and just tried our hardest to stay positive. That wasn't easy as he told us that we may not have got to this pregnancy in time and it would likely miscarry too. It was all I could think of as I prepared myself for another disappointment. A few weeks later a scan showed a little heart beating away and we could have screamed from the rooftops. I was in total disbelief. I had convinced myself that we would be going through the heartache all over again.

As we had only ever had negative experiences of scans and pregnancies, I had nothing positive to draw from and had got myself completely worked up with anxiety. I have to admit, the minute I left that scan I worried about what the next one would show, and this happened after almost every appointment to come. I felt it was never-ending and I couldn't focus on anything else day to day, but here I am having grown a baby to full term and some days I still can't believe it.

Someone told me that all the heartache would be worth it and at the time I didn't believe them, but without going through all of that I would have a different baby now and that doesn't bear thinking about.

THINKING ABOUT
GETTING PREGNANT?

Perhaps you are reading this book because you are planning to try for a baby in the near future, or you might have sadly experienced pregnancy losses and feel ready to start trying again. Either way, it is brilliant to have you here with me.

Whatever stage you are at, I want you to remember that your body is amazing. After miscarrying, at times I felt so angry towards my body for failing me, for not doing what it was supposed to. I lost trust in it, which felt truly awful and quite a scary place to be. It took some time, but once I started to trust my body again and not work against it, I felt this immense sense of pride over it. Not only had it been pregnant multiple times, but it had also recovered from losing those pregnancies, restored things, and rebalanced my hormones time and time again. It was then that I truly realized that we were on the same team.

My area of expertise is fitness, but preparing for pregnancy is about so much more than how much exercise it is deemed safe to do. It is important to consider your lifestyle and mental state too. How much sleep are you getting? How stressed are you? Are you nourishing your body? After all, you want your body to grow a human, so it needs to feel ready and safe to do so. You may not need to make drastic changes to your lifestyle, but keep checking in with yourself to make sure you are not overdoing it and that your body is happy.

A lot of women ask me whether they need to stop exercising when they are trying to conceive and that is absolutely

> YOU WANT YOUR BODY TO GROW A HUMAN, SO IT NEEDS TO FEEL READY AND SAFE TO DO SO.

not the case, unless you have received medical advice to the contrary. Staying active is great for you, but what is important is finding that balance between an active and healthy lifestyle and over-exercising, which can look different for everyone (see box, opposite). You'll come to realize that every answer in the pre- and postnatal world is accompanied by a disclaimer saying that everyone is different and every 'body' is different. This can be frustrating to hear when you just want an answer, but it couldn't be more true at this time in our lives.

TRYING TO CONCEIVE

Trying for a baby can cause anxiety, not least because it's probably one of the first times in our lives when we don't have control and can't plan things exactly as we would like. We don't know exactly when we will conceive, and the waiting game can feel never-ending. I felt an overwhelming sense of 'losing time' every month that I wasn't pregnant, which I know is crazy because there is no right time, but it can become all you think about.

It is incredibly important to keep communicating with your partner throughout this time and make sure that you are both on the same page. Your partner is likely to be feeling some of the same emotions as you. That two-week wait in-between your ovulation window

TOO MUCH **EXERCISE?**

Over-exercising can have many negative impacts on the body, including fatigue, slow recovery between sessions, and injury. It can also result in inhibiting the production of vital hormones such as progesterone, needed to sustain a healthy pregnancy. In fact, did you know that because progesterone is the precursor to cortisol, when cortisol levels increase, progesterone levels can decrease? This is exactly what you don't want happening when you're trying for a baby.

Try not to worry about your body being stressed – that is no good for anyone – but simply look at your exercise regime for that week and ask yourself whether your body has enough time to recover. If you love your higher-intensity workouts, try to keep them to one or two per week rather than every day.

and your period coming (or not) can be really tough, with days on end spent symptom-spotting and second-guessing everything. No matter whether it is your first month trying to conceive or you've been trying for a while, don't underestimate the stress that this can put on you and your partner.

As early pregnancy symptoms can be similar to those of an impending period, it's near impossible to tell whether you're pregnant. Try to keep busy and not think about it too much until your period is

> IT IS INCREDIBLY IMPORTANT TO KEEP COMMUNICATING WITH YOUR PARTNER THROUGHOUT THIS TIME.

due, though I know that is easier said than done. Don't spend money on umpteen overpriced pregnancy tests, only for your period to arrive bang on time. Try to wait until you are a little overdue at least. I talk from experience as I spent far too much on pregnancy

tests and even once accidentally signed up for a subscription delivery of them, so they kept turning up at my door. Doing a test days after you think you conceived might feel like a good idea, but it is highly unlikely to show a positive result at this time. I know it is very easy for me to say these things in hindsight, but it really did send me crazy. For this pregnancy I finally learnt my lesson and waited the long two weeks before I did a test.

KNOW YOUR CYCLE

When you are trying to conceive, it is worth getting to know your monthly cycle. There are apps that you can download to help you log data, so that you can track when your ovulation window falls and, more importantly, look out for other signs at that time.

Be mindful that not everyone's cycle is the textbook 28 days, and it can change from month to month – mine certainly did. When I started logging my cycle, I found it interesting to note the patterns with my moods and hormone surges. I may be a bit geeky about these things,

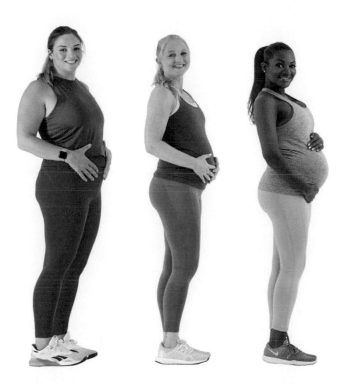

but I feel empowered when I know what is going on with my body and why it makes me feel a certain way.

Getting your period when you're trying for a baby can really knock you sideways, and you start seeing pregnant women everywhere – it can feel like a really cruel nightmare. Every time we went through a miscarriage or had a negative pregnancy test result, I felt disappointed and like I had been punched in the stomach, but I learnt to quickly turn it around and tell myself, "Okay, this time it wasn't meant to be, but now I have another two weeks before ovulation comes round again and in that time I am going to nourish and look after my body." I encouraged George to do the same, so that we had the best possible chance next time. Don't forget that it takes two people to make a baby.

Even if everything was aligned and you managed to catch ovulation at exactly the right time, there is still only around a 30 per cent chance of conceiving, which is much lower than I had realized. So don't beat yourself up if this month didn't work for you; it doesn't mean you have fertility problems. It is normal for it to take up to a year to conceive so, as hard as it feels, patience is the key. You've got this! Your turn is coming!

I'M PREGNANT!
NOW WHAT?

Seeing those two lines appear on a pregnancy test brings a whole host of emotions, whether you've longed to see them or it is a total shock. The first time for us was a complete and utter surprise. I gasped out loud, stared at the result window in disbelief for a while, and rushed to the shop to buy another two tests just to make sure. Although a positive result is a positive result, no matter how faint the line may be, women do an average of three pregnancy tests to confirm the result!

I jumped straight into action stations – I had to inform the doctor immediately, right? I made an appointment to see my GP the very next day and told him I was pregnant, to which he said, "Great, congratulations" and told me I could refer myself to a maternity unit – and that was that! I had expected another test to be done at the very least, and maybe fireworks to go off or something, but, no, he trusted the result of my test so off I went.

It felt pretty underwhelming going home knowing nothing more than what that home test had told us, so in subsequent pregnancies I trusted in the results and contacted the maternity unit straight away to register with them.

A JUMBLE OF FEELINGS

Mixed feelings are normal in the early stages. Even if you are delighted to be pregnant, there may also be anxiety, fear, and other negative thoughts going through your mind. Whether it is your first pregnancy or fifth, let's not forget what a huge life change it is to have a baby and it can take a while to get your head around it.

After seeing a positive test result, I felt totally consumed by it and my brain couldn't focus on much else for a while. I quickly calculated how many months pregnant I would be by my friend's wedding, when I was going to be her bridesmaid, and by Christmas – I sort of mapped out the next nine months within a matter of hours! All of a sudden, everything had changed. I kept going back to stare at all three of the pregnancy tests just to check. There they were, still saying "pregnant". I didn't always feel elated, though, and I think it's important to remember that a sudden rush of hormones can contribute to all sorts of feelings. It is good to prepare yourself for that and practise self-care.

For this pregnancy, I told George immediately. In fact, I woke him up at 6am and shoved the pregnancy test stick in front of him! The poor guy got a bit of a fright and didn't really know what

> WHETHER IT IS YOUR FIRST PREGNANCY OR FIFTH, LET'S NOT FORGET WHAT A HUGE LIFE CHANGE IT IS TO HAVE A BABY, AND IT CAN TAKE A WHILE TO GET YOUR HEAD AROUND IT.

to say, but I could see the multiple emotions rushing through his brain. We just gave each other a look as if to say, "Okay, here we go again", but we both had hope. He kept saying that he felt

like this one was the one, and as much as I didn't want him to jinx our luck, he said we needed to stay positive and he was absolutely right!

SHARING THE NEWS

We didn't tell anyone the first few times we conceived. However, after going through all the heartache of the pregnancy losses, this time we decided to tell one or two best friends and our immediate families at around seven weeks, just so we had a little more support and so that they knew what was going on. I personally found it really helpful to be able to talk about it, to let them know how I was feeling, or how appointments had gone, because of course we had a fair few of them this time before the all-important 12-week scan, and each one filled me with anxiety.

You may not want to share the news before the 12-week scan, but confiding in one or two people can provide much-needed support. It gives you that option to talk to someone else, other than your partner, about your pregnancy if you need to, or someone to back up your stories when you're trying to get out of social situations. Being newly pregnant at Christmas was tricky – I definitely needed that back-up to help me get out of drinks parties!

If you're feeling anxious or over-whelmed about things, it can often help to talk to someone who has been through it recently or a family member that knows you and how your mind works. I had one of each and was very grateful for their listening ears.

PREGNANCY SYMPTOMS

Some women say they know they are pregnant even before they see a positive result on a pregnancy test, but the majority of women don't get any symptoms immediately, and that in itself can cause anxiety. Be reassured that it is very normal for symptoms not to appear for a few weeks and that everyone experiences them differently.

My first symptom was my breasts growing and becoming very tender, but perhaps I was more aware of this because I have lived my whole life with a pretty flat chest. Some women start to feel nauseous or fatigued very soon after testing positive; some won't experience these symptoms until weeks six or seven, and some lucky ones never will at all. All of these variations are perfectly normal, so try not to compare your symptoms to anyone else because there isn't a 'one rule fits all' when it comes to pregnancy.

If you do have morning sickness, you will soon realize that it doesn't only happen in the morning. Carry snacks with you at all times because often an empty stomach can aggravate your symptoms, and through trial and error you will be able to figure out which snacks you can stomach best.

Every person under the sun will tell you to eat ginger biscuits or drink ginger tea if you say you have morning sickness, but unfortunately that doesn't work for everyone. For me it was crisps, any flavour at any time of day, so I stocked up the cupboard and made sure to carry some in my bag wherever I went, just in case.

YOU MAY NOT WANT TO SHARE THE NEWS
BEFORE THE 12-WEEK SCAN, BUT CONFIDING
IN ONE OR TWO PEOPLE CAN PROVIDE
MUCH-NEEDED SUPPORT.

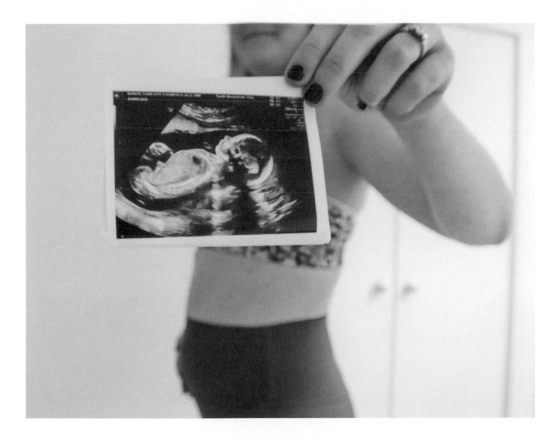

If you were an avid gym go-er before pregnancy and suddenly get hit by morning sickness and fatigue, you are quite likely to have to adjust your routine.

MAKING ADJUSTMENTS

If you start to feel sick or exhausted, and you find that exercise falls further and further down your to-do list, that is okay. Whilst it is safe to continue to exercise in the first trimester, now is probably not

YOU WILL BE ABLE TO GET YOURSELF BACK INTO SOME FORM OF EXERCISE SOON... REMEMBER, YOUR BODY IS DOING SOMETHING SO SPECIAL AND IMPORTANT; THIS IS NOT YOU BEING LAZY!

the time to be pushing through a workout if you feel awful. Find activities that might help alleviate some of your symptoms – maybe going for a walk in the fresh air or for a gentle swim. If you find that nothing helps, perhaps what your body needs is some downtime right now. Rest when you can, grab a quick afternoon nap here and there, and do whatever you need to get through the day.

When you can't use exercise as a form of release, you may find it a bit of a mental struggle at times, and I can totally empathize with that. It is important to keep reminding yourself why you are feeling so lethargic – that tiny baby is taking all the energy it needs to grow and not leaving you with any spare. You will be able to get yourself back into some form of exercise soon, so try not to add guilt on top of everything else you're feeling right now. Remember, your body is doing something so special and important; this is not you being lazy!

A large majority of women will start to feel better around 12–14 weeks, having less sickness and a bit more energy, at the start of the second trimester. So there is usually an end in sight and it can be really helpful to keep reminding yourself of that on those down days.

HOW I TRIED TO **COMBAT NAUSEA**

Here are some of the things that I found helpful for combatting nausea in the first trimester. They may not work for you, but are worth giving a go because, let's face it, when you feel that never-ending nausea you will try anything!

- **Eat something (anything):** I ate as soon as I got up in the morning. I learnt the hard way that an empty stomach was asking for trouble.
- **Cold grapes:** I would go into panic mode if I didn't have grapes in the fridge or the freezer; something about how easy they were to eat – with no preparation needed – was appealing to me.
- **Adding flavour to my water:** I knew I needed to stay hydrated as that really helped, but some days even the thought of drinking water made me gag, so a tiny drop of elderflower cordial would do the trick for me. Try a squeeze of lemon or cucumber or mint if you prefer.
- **Crisps:** I have a sweet tooth through and through, but strangely during pregnancy the one thing that would be guaranteed to ease the nausea for me was savoury, especially crisps. Although anything salty and crunchy would do – breadsticks, crackers, cheese straws. I wasn't too fussy, as long as there was plenty of them.

- **Swimming:** One day I turned up at the gym and couldn't face a workout so thought I'd give the pool a go and see how it went. To my surprise I felt free from nausea. Maybe it was the cool water – I'm not sure – but it worked well for me.
- **Driving with the windows down**: Even though it was mid-winter and freezing cold, that fresh air blowing right in my face really helped.
- **Afternoon naps:** I know not everyone is able to steal a cheeky 40-minute nap in the working day, and I felt guilty for doing it on some days because I felt like I should be doing something more productive with my time, but I felt better afterwards. Just 30–40 minutes, though, because any longer and I would often feel more tired when I woke up and then struggle to get going again.

If you happen to be one of the lucky ones who doesn't get any nausea or morning sickness, then don't wish for it. I know that in the first few weeks I was desperate for nausea as some sort of sign that something was happening in there, but just because you feel great doesn't mean that something is wrong. Some women just don't experience sickness, so if this is you, then don't panic.

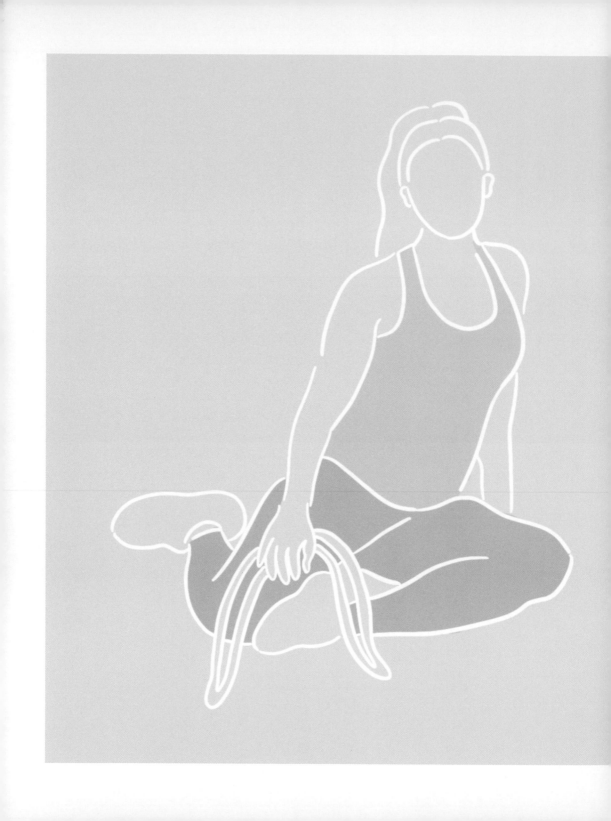

WARM UP & COOL DOWN

Gentle stretches

In this section you will find gentle exercises, suitable for all stages of pregnancy, for before and after your workout. They can be a relaxing workout in themselves on those days when you'd rather stretch than do a full workout.

WARM UP

There are 10 warm-up stretches in this section – choose four that target the muscles you will be exercising. I urge you not to skip them, even if you are short of time, as warming up gently eases you into your workout and prepares your body for what's to come.

REPEAT SET X 3

1. Arm circles

Move your arms in a circular motion, 10 forwards and 10 backwards.

2. Crab walks

Keeping the knees soft, and your weight over your heels, step sideways leading with your knee. The lower down the leg the band, the more difficult it is. Do 10 repetitions.

3. Banded glute bridges

Push your weight through your heels, keeping the tension in the band with your knees. Move your hips up and down 10 times. In the second and third trimester, it may feel more comfortable to do this exercise with your back leaning on the edge of the sofa.

4. Cat cow

Exhale as you round your spine and tuck your chin to your chest. Inhale as you look up to create the opposite curve. Do 5–10 repetitions.

5. Marching

Moving opposite arm to leg, march on the spot for a count of 10.

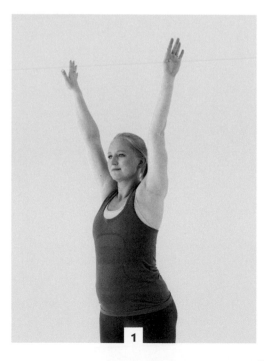

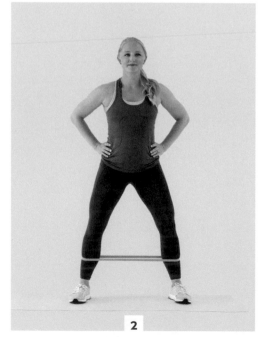

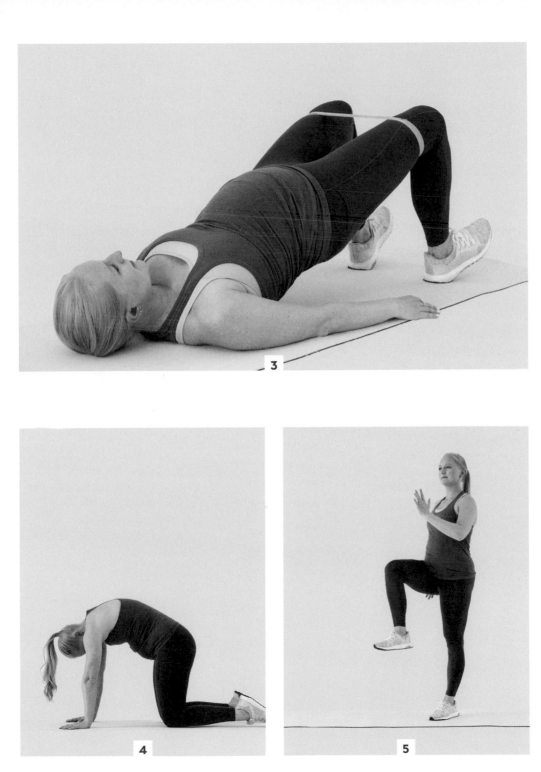

WARM UP

There are many good reasons to warm up: it gets your body ready for exercise by raising its temperature and encourages more blood flow to the muscles, reducing the risk of you feeling sore and getting injured.

REPEAT SET X 3

1. Kneeling clam

Keep your weight evenly spread across both hands as you lift one leg to the side using the glutes. Do 10 repetitions each side.

2. Thoracic twists

Thread one arm underneath your body, aiming for your ear to move towards the floor. Bring your arm back through and open your chest as you reach up to the ceiling. Do 5 repetitions.

3. Belly breathing

Do this on all-fours or seated. As you inhale, relax your core and let your bump come out as far as it can without moving your back. As you exhale, gently engage your core, hugging your bump up towards your spine, again keeping your back still. Inhale and exhale slowly to counts of 4.

4. Banded squat

Keeping your chest up and knees wide, push against the band on the way up and down. Do 10 repetitions.

5. Banded floor clam

Keep your knees bent and stacked above each other. With your ankles together, lift your top knee up. Do 10 repetitions each side.

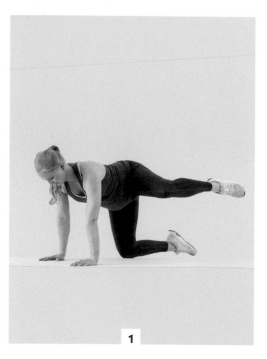

1

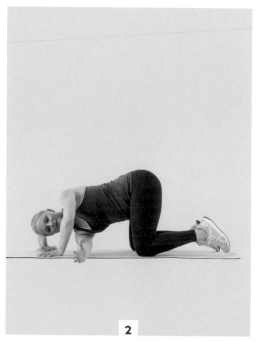

2

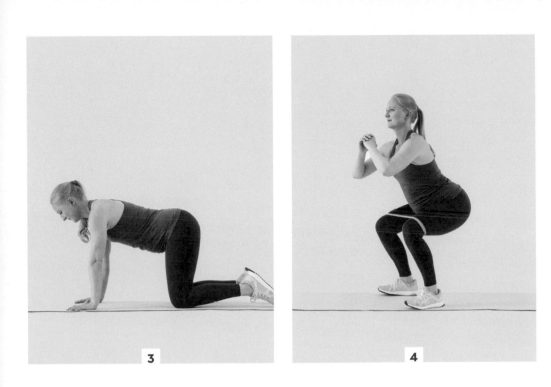

3

4

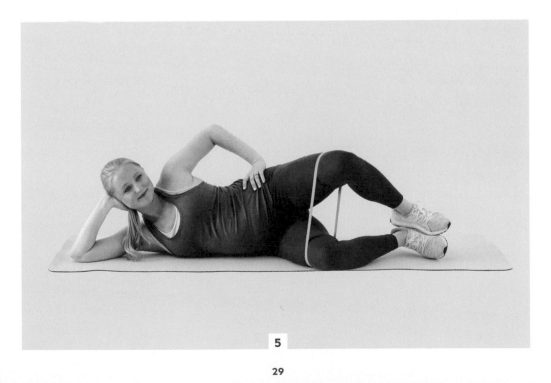

5

COOL DOWN

It's important to stretch at the end of a workout, but the extra relaxin in your body during pregnancy (see page 72) means you need to be careful of over-stretching. Go into each stretch slowly and hold it where it feels good for you.

REPEAT SET X 3

1. Hip flexor

Go down on one knee. Keep your pelvis tucked under and lean forward just enough to feel the hip flexor and/or quad stretching. Hold for 20–30 seconds on each leg.

2. Forward fold

Stand with your legs wider than hip-width apart and keep your knees soft. Fold forwards and let your body hang and sway from side to side to allow your back and hamstrings to lengthen. Hold for 10–20 seconds.

3. Lateral stretch

Stand with your legs wider than hip-width apart and reach up and over to each side, holding each stretch for 10–20 seconds.

4. Across body stretch

Using one arm, pull the other one across the front of your body. You may have to move it up and down to find where it best stretches your shoulder and tricep. Hold for 10–20 seconds each side.

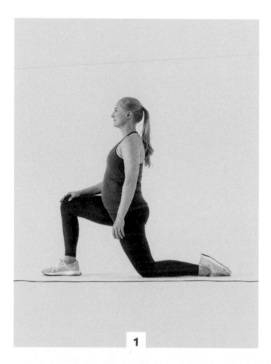

1

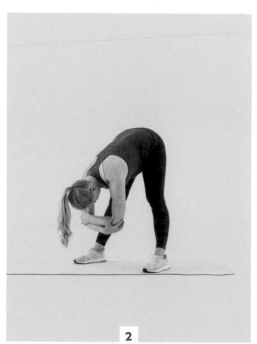

2

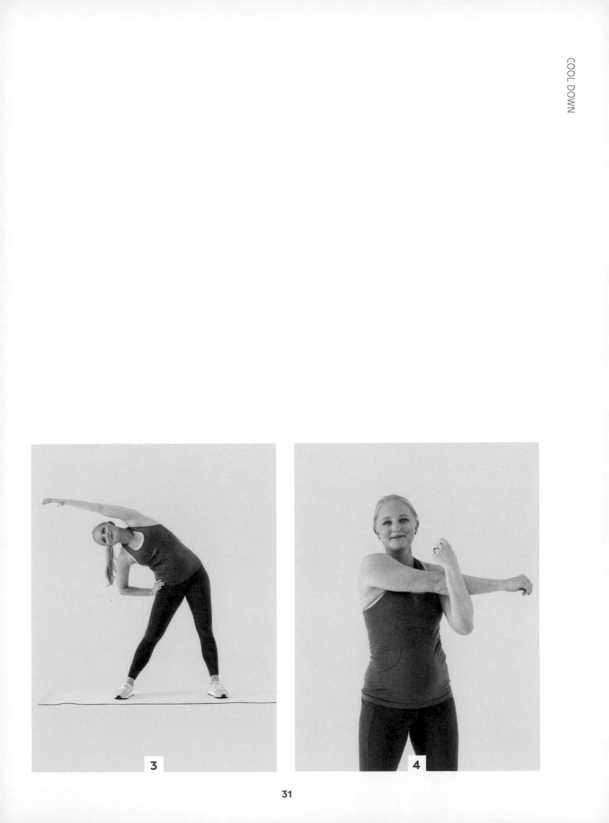

3

4

31

COOL DOWN

I know you may be short of time, but the longer you can spare to cool down the better. You can do stretching exercises even when you're not working out. They are great for helping with those tight muscles as your bump gets bigger and you start to feel a little achy.

REPEAT SET X 3

1. Tricep stretch

Reach down your spine with one hand as you gently pull the elbow with your other hand. Hold this for 10 seconds before switching to the other side.

2. Chest stretch

Clasp both hands together behind your back and, opening your chest, pull your hands away from your body. Look up for an extra stretch. Hold for 10–20 seconds.

3. Quad stretch

Holding on to something for extra balance if you need to, pull your foot up towards your bottom, trying to keep your knees together. Hold for 10 seconds. Repeat on the other leg.

4. Glute stretch

Sit tall and rest one foot over your knee. Lean forward just enough to feel the glute stretch in the bent leg. Hold for 10–20 seconds each side. As your bump grows, position the foot that is on the floor further away from you.

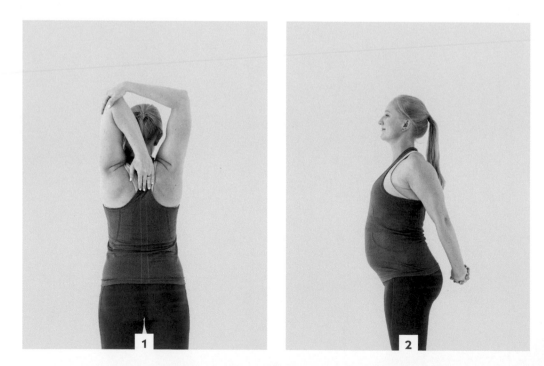

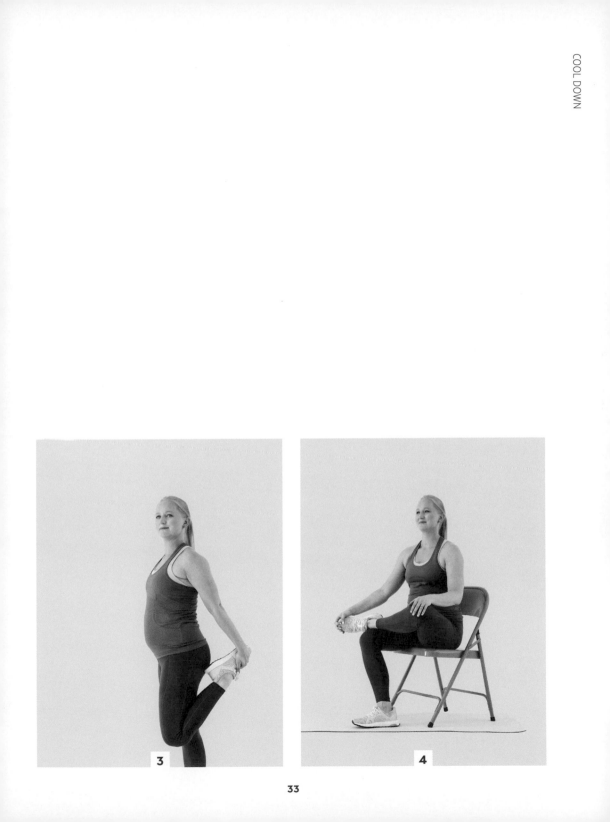

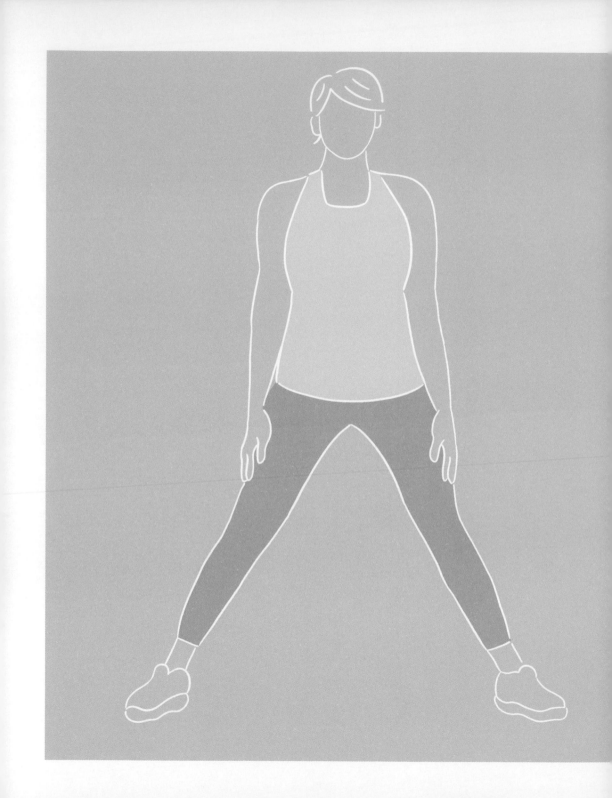

POSE DIRECTORY

Exercises to suit you

There are over 50 exercises to choose from in the directory, organized by lower body, upper body, and core workouts. Follow the step-by-step instructions and modify them as necessary depending on your stage of pregnancy.

LOWER BODY
EXERCISES

It is important to keep your lower body strong as it supports posture changes as your bump grows. A strong lower body can mean fewer aches and pains.

BODYWEIGHT
SQUAT

The squat is the foundation of many everyday movements. Perfecting the posture will enable you to get up and down off the sofa with ease while holding a wriggly baby!

Stand with your knees just wider than hip-width apart (or as much as your bump needs).

Keep your chest up and your knees driving outwards throughout.

Inhale as you squat down, exhale on the way up, engaging your core where possible.

If you are using dumbbells, hold them on your shoulders throughout.

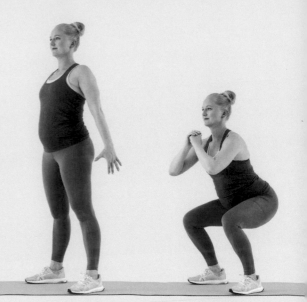

PULSING
SQUAT

This is like the bodyweight squat, above, but adding a pulse in at the bottom challenges your legs and glutes that little bit more.

Stand with your knees just wider than hip-width apart and if you are using dumbbells, hold them to your upper chest.

Keep your chest up and your knees driving outwards throughout.

Inhale as you squat down and pulse three times at the bottom of the squat.

Exhale a small breath in the pulse and a long breath on the way back up to standing.

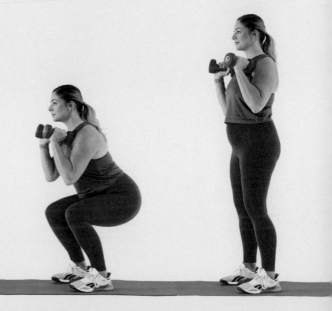

SUMO **SQUAT**

This is like a normal squat, but with the added weight of a dumbbell in front of your body, mimicking holding your baby.

Hold the dumbbell with two hands underneath your chin.

Stand with your knees just wider than hip-width apart (or as wide as your bump needs).

Keep your chest up and your knees driving out over your little toes throughout the exercise.

Inhale as you squat down and exhale on the way up.

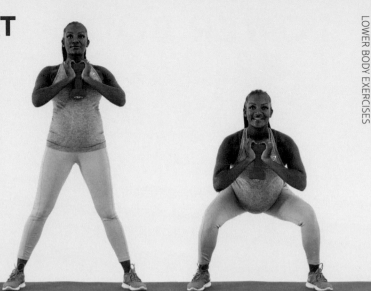

MAKE IT EASIER

For a lighter weight, hold one dumbbell with two hands instead.

SQUAT & **PRESS**

Adding a press into the squat movement will work your shoulders and upper back, but also activate your core.

Hold the dumbbells on your shoulders as you squat down.

As you exhale and stand, push both dumbbells straight up.

LOWER BODY EXERCISES

Movements like lunges help you to practise being off balance when bending down. Hold on to a table or chair for support if you feel you need it some days.

BACKWARD **LUNGE**

Always do the lunge backwards because it lessens the impact on your knees and it is usually easier to keep your balance this way. Alternate each leg.

Stand with your legs hip-width apart. Keep your chest up and shoulders relaxed throughout the exercise.

Inhale as you step backwards into the lunge. Aim to position both knees at a 90-degree angle. Your knee should not touch the floor, but hover just above it.

Exhale and step back up to standing.

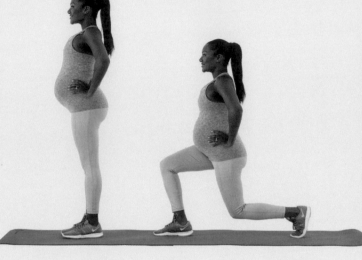

BALANCE **LUNGE**

In this lunge you bring your leg up in front you, requiring you to use your core muscles to balance.

Stand with your legs hip-width apart. Keep your chest up and shoulders relaxed throughout the exercise.

Inhale as you step backwards into the lunge. Aim to position both knees at a 90-degree angle. Your knee should hover just above the floor.

As you exhale to stand up, bring your knee up to a hold in front of you, then take it back into the next lunge.

Place your foot back on the ground in between each lunge if you need to.

Do all repetitions on one leg, then repeat for the other leg.

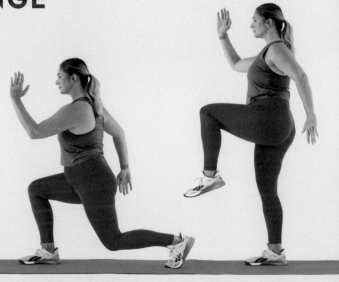

LUNGE & **CURL**

Adding a curl into the lunge creates a fuller movement, working the upper body alongside the lower body. Alternate each leg.

Stand with your legs hip-with apart. Hold the dumbbells down by your side.

Keep your chest up and shoulders relaxed throughout the exercise.

Inhale and curl the dumbbells up towards your shoulders as you step backwards into the lunge.

Aim to position both knees at a 90-degree angle. Your knee should not touch the floor, but hover just above it.

Exhale as you come up to standing again.

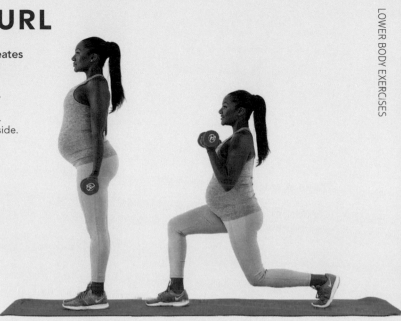

MAKE IT **HARDER**

Holding a dumbbell while you do the static lunge works the upper body too.

STATIC **LUNGE**

Use this instead of the backward lunge if you are feeling unsure about that movement due to pelvic girdle pain or lack of balance. It is effective for single leg strength.

Start with your legs split ready for a lunge movement.

Inhale and lower down into the lunge. Aim to keep your knees at a 90-degree angle. Your knee should not touch the floor, but hover just above it.

Keep your chest upright and your front knee pushed out over your little toe throughout the exercise.

Exhale as you come back up.

Repeat for the other leg.

LOWER BODY
EXERCISES

As well as more lunges, there's an emphasis on bending and lifting here – something you'll be doing a great deal of when you're a mum!

SIDE **LUNGE**

Exercises where we move side to side, rather than forwards and backwards, ensure we are strong in all directions. Alternate from side to side with this lunge.

Stand with your feet together and your arms by your sides.

Step into the lunge, keeping your weight in your heel and your hips pushed back.

Reach over towards the bent leg with your dumbbell. Keep the other leg straight.

Exhale as you come back to standing.

MAKE IT HARDER

Hold a dumbbell against the top of your chest.

STATIC **SIDE LUNGE**

This takes the impact out of a regular side lunge, so it is a good option if you are struggling with balance or pelvic girdle pain. It is a great exercise for when your bump gets heavier. Alternate from side to side with this lunge.

Start with your legs in a wide stance.

Inhale as you lean over one leg, with your weight in your heel and your hips pushed back.

Exhale as you come back up to standing in that wide stance.

MAKE IT EASIER

Lose the dumbbell and do this as a bodyweight lunge instead.

GOOD
MORNING

This strengthens your hamstrings, which are needed to support that posterior chain as the bump grows and your posture changes. Even when it is done with no weights, this is a very effective exercise.

Stand with your legs hip-width apart. Keep your knees soft, but not bent. Your legs should not be dead straight.

Cross your hands over your chest and keep your back straight as you push your hips backwards to lower your torso down towards the mat.

Keep your weight backwards over your heels. When you feel a tightening in your hamstring, exhale and start to come back up to standing, keeping your knees soft.

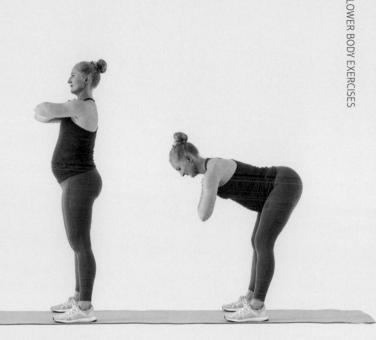

ROMANIAN
DEADLIFT (RDL)

A deadlift of any sort is vital for a mum-to-be to practise. It mimics the way you should bend over to pick your baby up out of the bath or the cot – these can be very awkward movements if you don't use the correct posture.

Stand with your legs hip-width apart. Keep your knees soft, but not bent. Your legs should not be dead straight. Hold the dumbbells in front of you.

Push your hips backwards, leaning your weight over your heels until you feel a tightening in your hamstrings. Don't go down any further than that.

Keep your spine in a neutral position by gazing down towards the mat.

Exhale and engage your core as you come back up to standing.

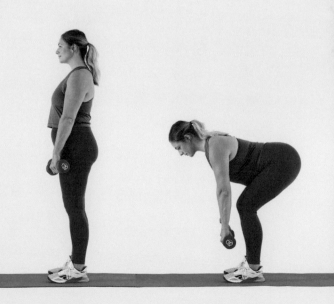

LOWER BODY EXERCISES

Strengthen those glutes! If they aren't strong, the lower back, pelvis, hip flexors, and knees over-compensate, which can put unnecessary strain on those areas.

SINGLE **RDL**

This is the same as a regular RDL (see page 41), but you focus on one leg at a time. The bent leg is there for balance – it should not do any work.

Stand with one leg bent and slightly behind you, but keep your knees in line with each other. Soften the front knee.

Hold your dumbbells down by your side. Push your hips back and keep your weight over the heel as you bend over, keeping your back in a neutral position.

Once you feel a tightening in your hamstring, exhale and gently come back up to standing.

Do all repetitions on one leg, then repeat on the other side.

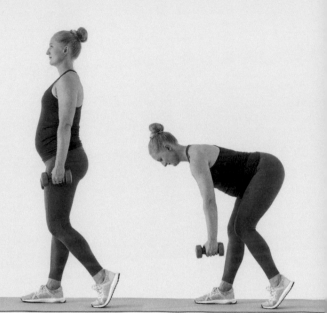

SUMO **DEADLIFT**

Deadlift is a way to pick something up off the floor, so this exercise is good preparation for babycare.

Start with your legs a little wider than you would for a squat, with your feet turned out ever so slightly. Hold the dumbbell(s) down in-between your legs.

Inhale as you lower down, pushing your knees out over your little toes and keeping your chest upright.

Exhale as you come back up to standing. Don't let your knees drop inwards as you do so.

Keep your neck in a neutral position, looking slightly ahead at the mat.

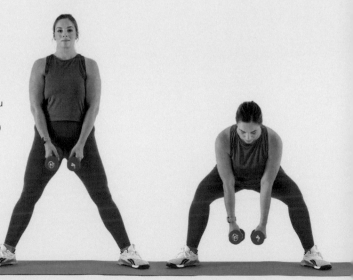

GLUTE
BRIDGE

It is important to keep your glutes nice and strong throughout pregnancy, and afterwards, so this is a great way to target them.

Lie on your back (see safety note below).

Push your weight through your heels only, and lift your hips until they are in line with your knees. Do not over-extend your back.

Squeeze your glutes at the top of the movement, before lowering back down again.

If you are using a dumbbell, hold it around your hips or upper leg.

Safety note: It is not advisable to stay lying on your back for long periods from the second trimester (see page 9). An alternative way to do these glute bridge exercises is to lean your upper back on the edge of the sofa, then lower your hips up and down towards the floor.

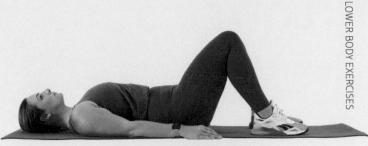

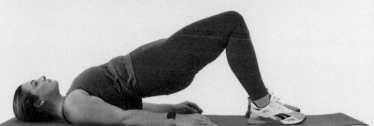

SINGLE
GLUTE BRIDGE

This single version has the added advantage of working your legs without having to maintain the balance you would while standing.

Lie on your back (see safety note above).

Keep one leg bent with your heel on the mat. Straighten the other leg.

Push your hips up through the heel of the working leg, being careful not to over-extend your back or let your hip drop to one side.

If you are using a dumbbell, hold it around your hips or upper leg.

Do all repetitions with one leg, then repeat on the other side.

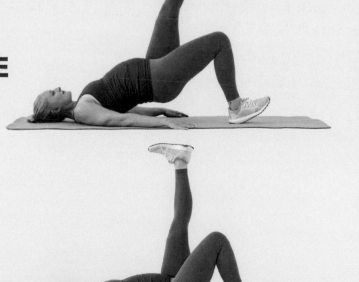

LOWER BODY
EXERCISES

We all love the idea of lying down to exercise but don't be fooled – there is little relaxing going on here. You'll feel the burn of the leg lifts and crunches pretty quickly.

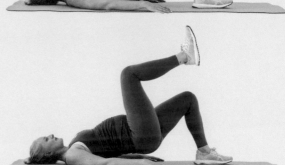

GLUTE BRIDGE
MARCH

By transferring your weight from one leg to the other you are working on your pelvic stability, which is important for supporting that growing bump.

Lie on your back (see safety note on page 43).

Keep one leg bent with your heel on the mat. Push your hips up through the heel of the working leg, being careful not to over-extend your back.

Alternate lifting one leg at a time, maintaining a bent knee. Take it slowly and keep your hips as still as possible throughout the exercise.

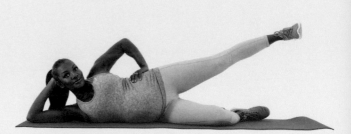

LYING
LEG RAISE

This is not as relaxing as it looks unfortunately, but it is brilliant for activating and isolating the glute muscles.

Lie on your side, with your head resting on your hand or flat on the floor.

Keep the underneath leg bent, with your top leg straight.

Maintain a flexed foot on the straight leg and raise it up to just above hip height and back down again to gently tap the floor, creating small pulse-like movements.

Repeat on the other side.

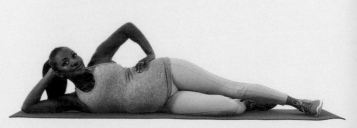

LYING
LEG CRUNCH

This is another glute-specific exercise and you can expect the burn to kick in quite quickly!

Lie on your side, with your head resting on your hand or flat on the floor.

Keep the underneath leg bent, with your top leg straight just above hip height.

Bend the upper leg in towards your bump and back out to the starting position.

Repeat on the other side.

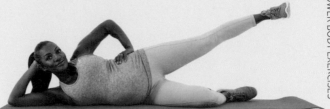

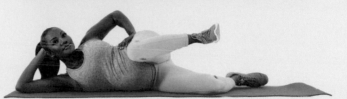

MODIFIED
BURPEE

You might be glad to know that burpees are discouraged as your bump grows too big, but there are ways to modify them so you can keep them in your exercise routine for as long as possible. Good news for some! This version takes out the impact aspect of burpees by replacing jumps with steps.

Stand with your legs wide apart to make it easier to reach the floor.

Place your hands on the mat in front of you and step back one foot at a time to a full plank (see safety note below).

Step forward one step at a time to bring yourself up to standing again.

Keep your back as straight as possible throughout and lower your bum before standing up to avoid hunching your back and causing discomfort further down the line.

Safety note: From the second trimester onwards, or if you find a full plank position too difficult, drop your knees to the mat.

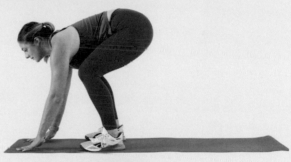

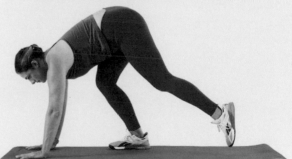

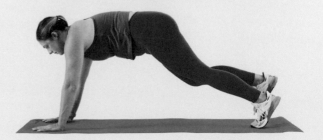

UPPER BODY
EXERCISES

It will be no surprise to you that you'll be needing to do a lot of lifting once your baby is here, so it is so important to have a good base of upper body strength.

REVERSE
TABLE TOP DIP

This exercise works almost every part of your body, and as the bump gets bigger, you'll have more and more to lift so it will work it all even harder.

Sit on the floor with your arms behind you and your hands facing slightly outwards to prevent discomfort in the wrists.

Keeping your arms straight, push your hips up off the ground. Only go as high as you feel comfortable, but no higher than a neutral spine, with your knees, hips, and shoulders in line. Do not over-extend your back.

Keep your weight in your heels to activate the glutes.

Slowly lower back down to a seated position.

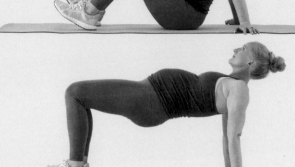

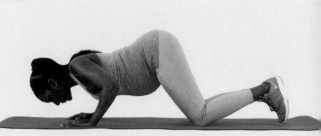

PRESS-UP

Many people find press-ups difficult, but don't let a bump put you off practising them. They are a great way to improve upper body strength, especially in the chest and shoulders.

Lower your knees to the mat, or stay in a full plank position if you are in the first trimester and feel that you can.

Keep your legs nice and wide so that you can stabilize your hips throughout the exercise.

Inhale and lower your chest down towards the mat.

Exhale and engage your core as you press your body back up to the start position.

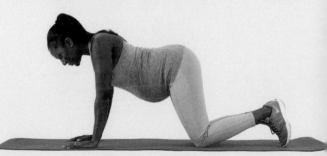

PRESS-UP &
SHOULDER TAP

This is like a regular press-up, but the addition of shoulder taps means you are adding in some bonus core work. Shifting your weight from side to side helps to build up your core stability around that growing bump.

As you come up from your press-up, carefully lift one arm to tap the opposite shoulder.

Then lift the other arm to tap the opposite shoulder.

Keep your hips as still as possible as you move your arms.

MAKE IT
HARDER

In the first trimester, you can do this in a full plank position if you feel your core can manage it.

ARM
RAISE

This incorporates upper body and core work in one go. It uses the upper body strength to balance on one arm at a time, and core strength to stabilize the hips as you go from side to side. It is important to pay close attention to your breathing.

In your half-plank position, keep your knees wide for stability.

Exhale and reach one arm up towards your ear, then inhale as you bring it back down.

Alternate your arms, making sure to engage your core as you lift them.

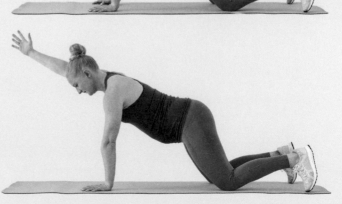

UPPER BODY
EXERCISES

Upper body strength is essential to protect your posture as your bump gets bigger and your growing breasts start to pull your shoulders forward.

PLANK
MARCH

As this exercise is intense on the shoulders, it really works to build strength for lifting. Keep your hips as still as possible to keep the core working hard.

Whether you are in a full plank (first trimester only) or on your knees, keep your legs nice and wide so you can stabilize your hips throughout the exercise.

One arm at a time, inhale as you lower down on to your elbows.

Exhale and engage your core as you push back up onto your hands.

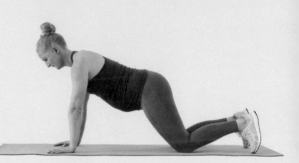

ALTERNATING
SHOULDER PRESS

Just like a regular shoulder press, but you are raising one arm at a time so that when one arm rests the other is working.

Stand with your feet hip-width apart and hold the dumbbells on your shoulders.

Exhale as you push one dumbbell up, straightening your arm.

Inhale as you bring it back down to your shoulder.

Repeat on the other side and continue alternating.

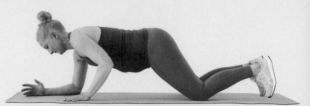

NARROW
SHOULDER PRESS

You won't be lifting your baby up over your head 10 times in a row, hopefully, but this movement will help to prepare you for the amount of lifting you will be doing. You can never be too prepared!

Stand with your feet hip-width apart.

Hold the dumbbells on your shoulders, with your fingertips facing your neck.

Exhale and engage the core as you press both dumbbells above your head, keeping your elbows tucked in.

Inhale as you bring both arms back to the start position.

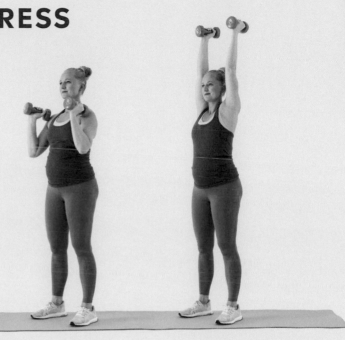

WIDE
SHOULDER PRESS

This movement is very similar to the narrow shoulder press, above, but with the wide positioning of the arms it also engages the upper back, which is key to maintaining a good posture.

Stand with your feet hip-width apart.

Hold the dumbbells just above your shoulders with your elbows in a wide position and fingertips facing forwards.

Exhale and engage the core as you press both dumbbells up and towards each other.

Inhale as you bring them back down, keeping your elbows wide.

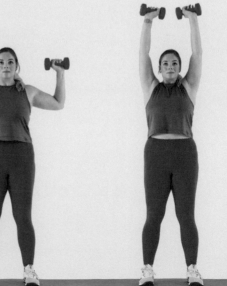

UPPER BODY
EXERCISES

You might find there are some days when you're lacking in energy and want to use lighter weights – that is okay and very normal. You're still working out!

CURL & **PRESS**

This is exactly the same as the regular shoulder press, but with a bicep curl in-between, bringing more arm muscles into the exercise.

Stand comfortably with your feet hip-width apart and keep your knees soft for balance.

Exhale and engage your core as you curl the dumbbells up towards your shoulders and then up above your head, rotating your hands as you do so.

Inhale as you bring them back down to the start position.

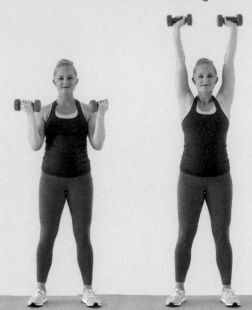

BENTOVER **ROW**

Any rowing movement is brilliant for working the upper back, which is key to keeping a good posture during pregnancy and afterwards.

Stand with your legs hip-width apart. Keep your knees soft, but not bent. Your legs should not be dead straight.

Start with the dumbbells in front of your body at about knee height.

Push your hips back with your weight in your heels and lower your chest down to face the mat.

Keeping your spine in a neutral position, exhale and pull the dumbbells up towards your body.

Squeeze your upper back muscles by bringing your shoulder blades towards each other. Inhale as you lower the weights.

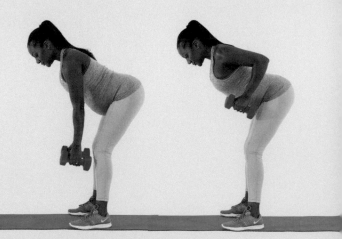

SINGLE
BENTOVER ROW

Like the standard bentover row, opposite, but you are working one side at a time. In some instances, this will allow you to opt for a heavier weight if you wish to.

Hold your dumbbell in one hand. Lean forward with the other hand resting either on your front leg or against a stable chair.

Keep the other leg out behind you in a straight and stable position.

Keep both hips facing forward, making sure not to open your hip angle as you go through the exercise.

Exhale as you pull the dumbbell up towards your body, squeezing your upper back at the top of the movement.

Inhale as you gently release the weight back down.

Repeat on the other side.

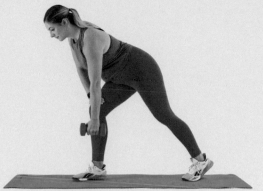

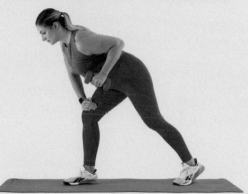

RENEGADE ROW

This is another great exercise for working the upper back muscles, but this time in a plank position so that you activate your core as well.

Position yourself either in a full plank (first trimester only) or in a half-plank, keeping your legs in a wide stance to help stabilize your hips.

Rest your hands on your dumbbells, with your shoulders directly above your hands.

Exhale as you bring one dumbbell up towards your rib cage, keeping your hips as still as possible.

Inhale as you lower it back down to the mat, then repeat on the other side.

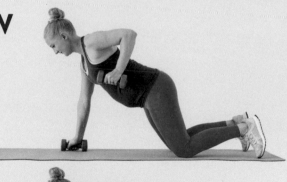

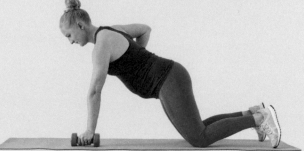

UPPER BODY
EXERCISES

It is an old wives' tale that pregnant women should not lift anything, but even so, we do need to be strong if we want to prove them wrong!

UPRIGHT **ROW**

This exercise really isolates the upper back muscles, which is important to help you stand nice and tall when your newfound posture wants you to hunch over.

Stand with your legs hip-width apart and your knees slightly soft.

Hold the dumbbells against your upper thighs.

Exhale and engage your core as you lift both dumbbells up towards your chin, with your elbows wide.

Engage your upper back at the top of the exercise, but be mindful not to shrug your shoulders.

Inhale as you lower the dumbbells back down again and bring your elbows in close to your body.

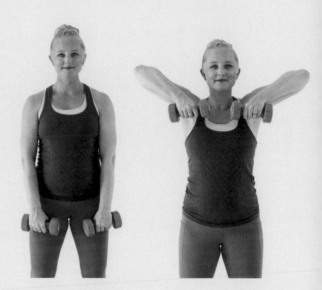

BICEP **CURL**

As the name suggests, this exercise isolates the bicep. This is one of the muscles that is used to cradle a baby, so the stronger it is before your baby arrives, the more comfortable those holds will be.

Stand with your legs hip-width apart and your knees slightly soft.

Start by holding the dumbbells against your upper thighs, with your palms facing out.

Exhale and engage your core as you bend at the elbow, bringing the dumbbells up towards your shoulders. Keep your shoulders relaxed and try not to shrug them.

Inhale as you lower the dumbbells back down again.

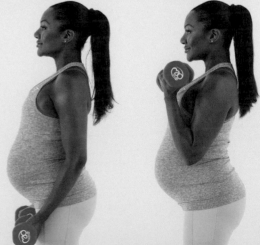

LATERAL **RAISE**

Lifting your arms up to the side like this is tougher than it looks and really works both the shoulders and the upper back.

Stand up straight with your shoulder blades engaged, your legs hip-width apart, and your knees slightly soft.

Start with the dumbbells down by your sides.

Exhale and engage your core as you raise the dumbbells up to the side to shoulder height, and no further.

Don't shrug your shoulders as you lift the dumbbells – keep a long and relaxed neck.

Inhale as you bring the dumbbells down again.

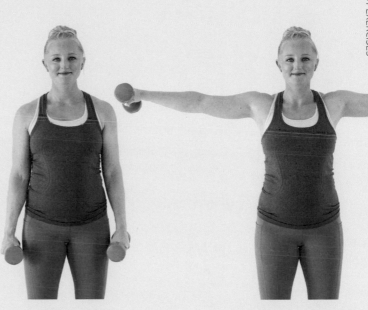

FRONTAL **RAISE**

A similar exercise to the lateral raise, above, but lifting the weights in front of you engages the front of your body rather than your back muscles.

Stand with your legs hip-width apart, with your knees slightly soft.

Hold the dumbbells in front of you at the top of your thighs.

Inhale and engage your core as you lift the dumbbells up to shoulder height.

Don't shrug your shoulders as you lift the dumbbells – keep your neck long and relaxed.

Inhale as you lower the dumbbells.

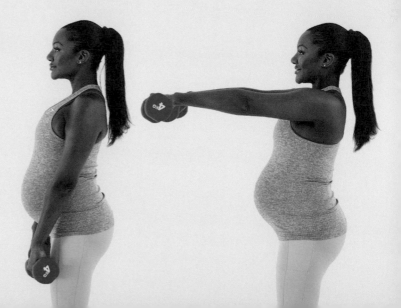

UPPER BODY
EXERCISES

Your baby is going to feel heavy pretty quickly, so let's get ahead of the game and make sure your arms are strong enough to lift and cuddle all day long with ease.

TRICEP **DIP**

This is another exercise that burns quicker than most, but it is important to be able to hold your own bodyweight and these tricep dips ensure just that.

Make sure the chair is stable and not going to slip before you start.

Place your hands on the chair with your fingertips facing you.

Keep your legs hip-width apart, or as wide as your bump needs.

Bend your arms to dip your hips down towards the floor, trying to keep your back close to the chair. Inhale as you do this.

Exhale as you push through your hands to come back up.

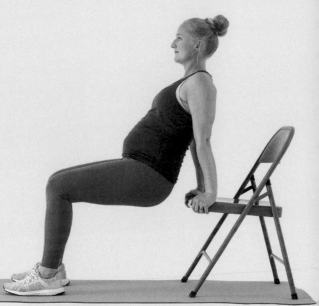

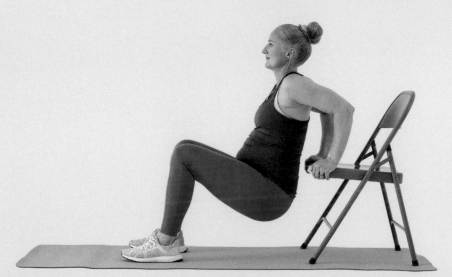

CHEST
PRESS

This complements the press
-up nicely, working the chest
and arm muscles but in
the opposite position.

In the first trimester, you can do
this lying on your back. From the
second trimester, use the glute
bridge position overleaf.

Start with the dumbbells above
your chest, with your arms
straight and your thumbs next
to each other.

Inhale as you lower your elbows
to the floor either side of you.

Exhale and engage your core
as you press the dumbbells up
to meet each other.

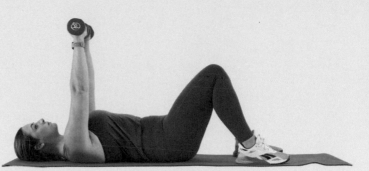

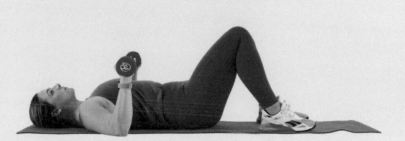

TRICEP
EXTENSION

The tricep is a small muscle
that tires easily, so don't be
surprised if this one burns
quickly! It's meant to.

Hold both dumbbells over your
head (or just use one if you want
to make it easier).

Keep your elbows positioned
close to your ears throughout.

Bend at the elbows, bringing
the dumbbells down towards
your upper back.

Exhale as you bring them back
up to the starting position.

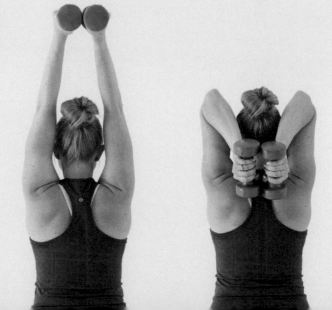

UPPER BODY
EXERCISES

Although these exercises work the chest and arms, the glutes get to join in too. Not only that, but with the correct breathing the core plays a part, making them very effective full-body exercises.

GLUTE BRIDGE
CHEST PRESS

This exercise is a chest press for the second and third trimesters to avoid you lying on your back for too long (see page 9). It also has the added benefit of activating your glutes as well as working your upper body.

Get into a glute bridge position (see page 43).

Hold the dumbbells out to the side, fingertips facing inwards. Inhale as you bend them and bring your elbows down towards the mat, and exhale as you push them up, straightening your arms and bringing the dumbbells together.

Inhale as you slowly bring the dumbbells back down again.

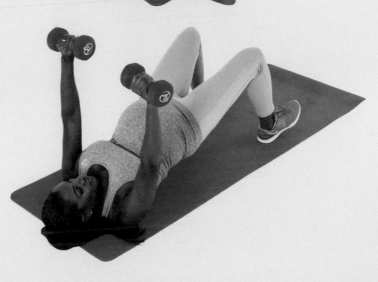

CHEST
FLYE

This exercise is excellent for really isolating the pectoral muscles, but with the correct breathing techniques the core can be involved too – a nice bonus!

In the first trimester, you can continue to do your chest flyes lying on your back if you feel comfortable in that position. Otherwise, and for the second and third trimesters, do the exercise below instead.

Lie on the mat with your legs bent.

Hold the dumbbells together above your chest with your fingers facing each other. Your arms should not be completely straight – keep them slightly bent at the elbow.

Lower both arms so the dumbbells move towards the floor.

Continue to keep your arms bent at the elbow and, as you exhale, lift and straighten them back up to meet in the middle.

GLUTE BRIDGE
CHEST FLYE

This exercise is a chest flye for the second and third trimesters to avoid you lying on your back for too long (see page 9). It also has the added benefit of activating your glutes as well as working your upper body.

Get into a glute bridge position (see page 43) and hold this for the entirety of the exercise.

Perform the chest flye in exactly the same manner as you would lying flat (see above).

MAKE IT HARDER

Try slowing down the movement and taking a count of three on the way down and the way up.

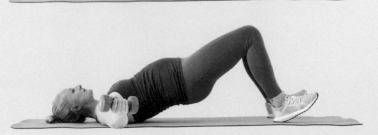

57

CORE EXERCISES

Even though those six-pack muscles are far from visible, it is more important than ever to keep the core muscles strong to support your growing bump.

SIDE PLANK

A side plank exercise activates and works the oblique muscles, which help to support your bump as it grows.

In the first trimester, start with your knees on the mat and gradually lift up to your feet, with one foot in front of the other for balance.

In later trimesters, or if you don't fancy the full plank, drop one or both knees to the mat (see below) to take a little pressure off your core.

Keep your hips as straight as you can, trying not to let your torso drop down towards the mat.

Repeat on the other side.

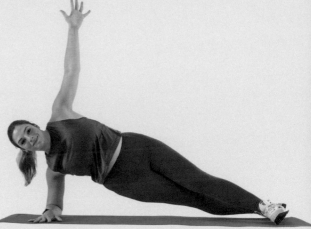

SIDE PLANK TWIST

This is the same as the regular side plank, above, but the twist movement challenges your core muscles that bit more.

Hold your side plank position, keeping your hips high throughout.

Bring your raised arm down and twist it under your body.

If you notice any doming in your core, make sure you are bending both knees, and exhaling to engage your core as you twist gently.

Repeat on the other side.

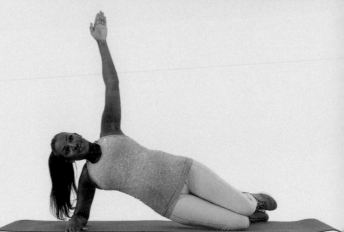

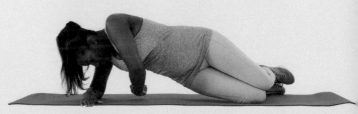

SIDE PLANK
DIP

The extra movement provided by the dip works your core a little harder, as well as your upper body.

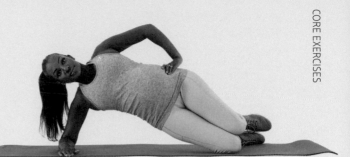

Get into a side plank position (see opposite) and keep your hand either on your hip or straighten it above you.

Dip your lower hip down towards the mat as you inhale.

Exhale and engage your core as you lift your hip back up to a neutral position.

Repeat on the other side.

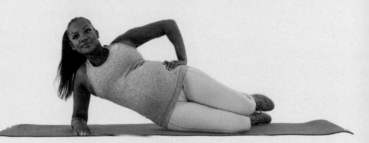

SIDE PLANK
CRUNCH

This challenging version in which you straighten your top leg requires strength and balance. If you have pelvic girdle pain, lower the top leg and just do the arm movements.

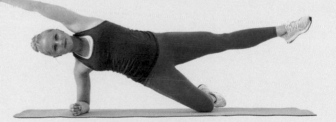

Get into a side plank position (see opposite).

Stretch your top arm and leg out in a straight line above your body.

Keeping your hips high, bring your arm and leg in so that your knee and elbow come towards each other. Make sure this crunch is above your body, not in front of it.

Exhale as you crunch in, and inhale as you extend your arm and leg out again.

Repeat on the other side.

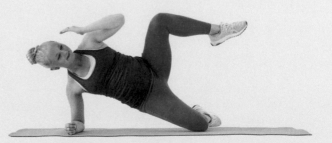

CORE EXERCISES

You'll be pleasantly surprised to discover how many ways you can still engage your core during pregnancy, especially with the use of your breath to help.

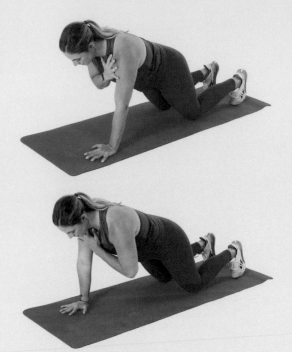

SHOULDER **TAP**

As you shift your weight from side to side, your core maintains stability and keeps you from falling. Take your time with this exercise.

Whether you are in a full plank (first trimester only) or a modified plank, engage your shoulder blades so your upper back isn't hunched.

Tilt the pelvis to keep your core engaged and spine in a neutral position.

Position your legs wider than your arms to help with core stability.

As you lift one hand to tap the opposite shoulder, try to keep your hips as still as possible, keeping your core engaged.

Exhale as you tap each shoulder.

BIRD **DOG**

The key to this exercise is good control and the correct breathing. It is very effective at getting the core to stabilize you and your bump.

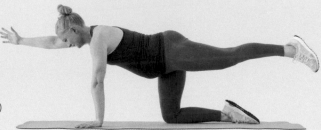

Start in a box position (see opposite page) on the mat with your knees and hands at hip- and shoulder- width apart.

Inhale as you lift opposite arm to opposite leg, creating a long straight line from fingertip to toe.

Exhale and engage your core as you bring your hand in to touch your knee.

Do all repetitions on the same side before switching.

If you are struggling with pelvic girdle pain or balance, keep your foot on the ground and slide it along the mat instead.

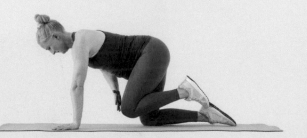

BELLY
BREATHING

I did this every day throughout pregnancy, even when I did no other exercise. It helped to calm my breathing down and activate my core. It is amazing to watch the bump going in and out, just proving how strong your core can still be. This is the all-fours position, but belly breathing can also be done in a lying or seated position.

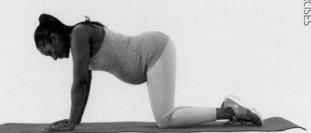

Position yourself on all fours, keeping your body in a relaxed state.

As you inhale, gently draw your bump and ribs in towards your spine and hold for 1–3 seconds.

Inhale as you let your tummy relax all the way out again.

If you start to feel dizzy at any point, take a break.

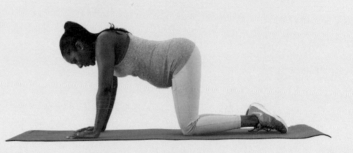

4-POINT
KNEE RAISE

This is challenging, so if you feel that you can't hold for the three seconds there is no harm in doing shorter holds. It is the breathing that is the important thing to practise here.

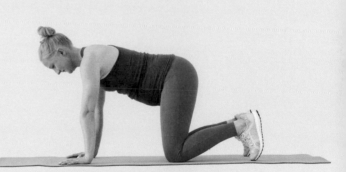

Start in a box position on the mat with your knees and hands at hip- and shoulder-width apart.

Keep your spine relaxed and in a neutral position.

Exhale while gently drawing your tummy in and lifting your knees off the mat only slightly.

Hold this for 1–3 seconds and lower back down to the mat with an inhale.

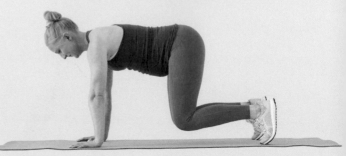

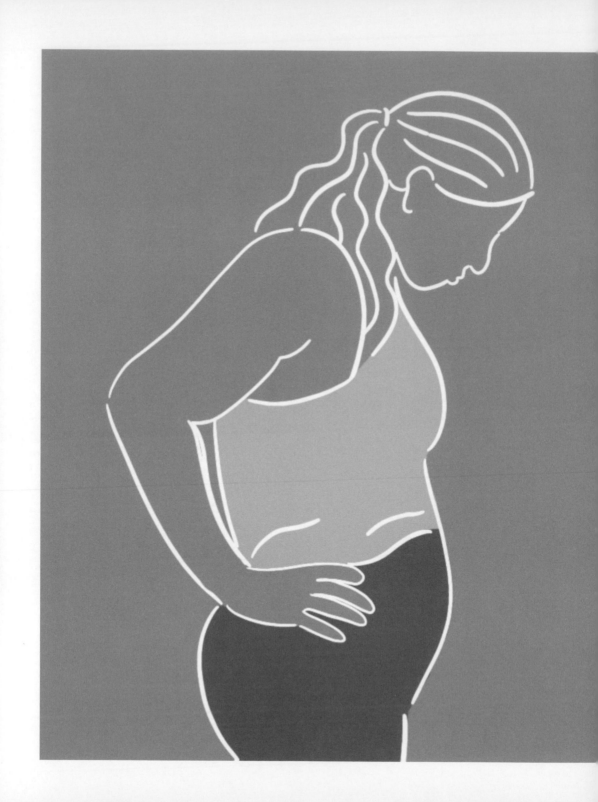

FIRST TRIMESTER
Weeks 1–12

This trimester starts with a positive pregnancy test result and ends with that all-important 12-week scan. Although there may be no tell-tale bump for a while, your baby develops rapidly in these first three months.

WHAT TO EXPECT IN
THE FIRST TRIMESTER

I felt like the first trimester went on forever – three months felt like six. I was anxious and because I had lots of extra appointments, I was always anticipating the next one. It was all I could think about. In hindsight, I lost far too many hours looking for answers on Google and Mumsnet and I would strongly advise you to try to stay away from both if you can.

If you have any pressing questions, ask your GP or midwife or another trusted source. It's so easy to get stuck down a rabbit hole Googling things such as, "If I cough too much, will I miscarry?" … and yes I did search that. I was quickly comforted by Google predicting my question, proving that clearly I wasn't the only crazy one! (And no you can't, in case you were wondering too.)

SYMPTOM CHECKING

I didn't have a bump for the whole of my first trimester. I thought I did and would send my Mum 'bump updates', to which she would politely get excited. Looking back, I realize I was sending her pictures of an ever so slightly bloated tummy post-lunch. My breasts were pretty sore and that was the symptom I was holding on to. I would check them for soreness throughout the day – I'm sure I looked a bit crazy doing this in the supermarket, but I didn't care!

One day I was certain they didn't feel sore anymore and my heart just sank, but of course I went straight to my trusty 'Dr Google', who reminded me that symptoms come and go. Sure enough, the very next day they were sore again. The mind can play such horrible

> IT'S SO EASY TO GET STUCK DOWN A RABBIT HOLE GOOGLING THINGS SUCH AS, "IF I COUGH TOO MUCH, WILL I MISCARRY?"

tricks on you when you're feeling that anxious.

We had an early scan at seven weeks, and when we heard the heartbeat I remember feeling like the luckiest girl in

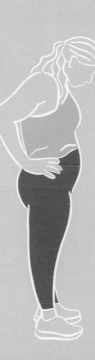

YOUR BABY AND BODY **IN THE FIRST TRIMESTER**

A lot happens during the first trimester, even though from the outside you may not look pregnant for a while yet.

The fertilized egg quickly divides into multiple layers of cells and implants itself into the wall of your womb, where it will carry on growing. Some women feel slight cramping at the time of implantation, but it's hard to pinpoint it and most women don't feel a thing, especially if they aren't looking out for it. The layers of cells will become an embryo, which is what your baby is called at this early stage.

During the first trimester the embryo will grow at a faster rate than at any other time in your pregnancy, so no wonder the tiredness kicks in! Your body is working so hard during this trimester.

By around six weeks, a heartbeat can usually be detected on an ultrasound scan and by 12 weeks your unborn baby's bones and muscles will have formed, as well as all of the organs. How incredible is that? Your body is doing all of that and most of your family and friends will still have no idea that you are pregnant!

the world. It was an internal ultrasound, so not the most pleasant of experiences, but I would have let it go on for hours just to keep seeing that heartbeat. That little flickering blob was all we had longed to see for the last year. We knew we weren't out of the woods yet though. Due to my miscarriage history and my over-active immune system we had a few more hoops to jump through before we could relax, but this was a big step in the right direction.

The next scan was on Christmas Eve and my anxiety leading up to it was

> WE SPENT ALL CHRISTMAS
> LOOKING AT THOSE SCAN
> PICTURES AND GRINNING
> FROM EAR TO EAR.

probably the worst. I was so nervous that our excitement from the last scan would be short-lived, but the lovely sonographer put her arm around me as she walked with us down the corridor.

There must have been something on my notes saying "severely anxious" or maybe she just saw it in my face. She very quickly turned the screen around and showed us our baby. This time it wasn't just a blob – we could see something that resembled a head and that heart was there still beating away, a bit faster this time. It was the best Christmas present we could have ever wished for. We spent all Christmas looking at those scan pictures and grinning from ear to ear.

BABY ON BOARD?

Like some women, you might want to wear a baby on board badge on public transport very early on in pregnancy to get that all-important seat. I don't blame you, especially if you're travelling in rush hour with morning sickness.

I shied away from wearing one because I was so nervous about doing anything to jinx the pregnancy – crazy, I know, but it made perfect sense to me at the time. I would actually find myself giving my seat to other women wearing their badge, through habit, and then

I COULDN'T BELIEVE I WAS FINALLY ONE OF THE WOMEN WEARING A BABY ON BOARD BADGE AND I HAPPILY ACCEPTED EVERY SEAT OFFERED TO ME!

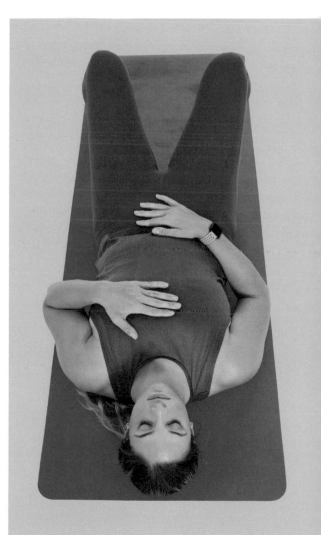

regret it when I had to stand up for the rest of my journey, knowing that I deserved that seat just as much. I didn't want strangers knowing I was pregnant before it even felt real to me, so I didn't wear my badge until around 20 weeks. I couldn't believe I was finally one of the women wearing a baby on board badge – it was my turn and I happily accepted every seat offered to me!

PELVIC PAIN

Pelvic Girdle Pain (PGP) is something that many women experience throughout pregnancy. One in five report symptoms of it and it most often starts in the second or third trimesters, but sometimes earlier, which is why it is in this section.

PGP used to be called SPD (Symphysis Pubis Dysfunction), but now it is the umbrella term for any pelvic pain. There are three pelvic joints – the symphysis pubis at the front and two sacroiliac joints at the back. A variety of factors contribute to PGP, including changes to the muscles and connective tissue surrounding those joints. If you have had a previous injury to the pelvic area, you may be more likely to have PGP.

Women experiencing PGP may have pain over the pubic bone, roughly level with their hips, across one or both sides of their lower back, but also around the perineum (the area between the vagina and anus), and it can commonly be felt down one or both thighs.

It can feel worse during or after a long walk, when going up and down stairs, when standing on one leg to get dressed, when getting in and out of a car, and when turning over in bed. Some women may be unable to walk much, let alone exercise, by the end of their pregnancy. I strongly recommend seeing a pelvic health physiotherapist (see page 203) if you have PGP. Treatment will depend on what is found in the assessment, but may include muscle release work and strengthening or stretching exercises. Crutches or support belts may be recommended. How your labour may be affected will be discussed and you will be given advice to help you.

Things that can help:
- Modifying movements and exercises – I found lunges painful, so I removed them from my workouts for a while.
- Sitting down to get dressed and put on shoes, to avoid having to stand on one leg.
- Keeping your legs together when turning in bed. Squeeze your legs together and your bottom muscles and use your upper body to help you roll.
- Taking smaller steps when walking.
- Taking the stairs one step at a time.
- Wearing supportive shoes, and not shoes that have a heel or are too flat.
- Avoiding sitting cross-legged.
- Using a plastic bag under your bottom to help you swivel in and out of your car

RED **FLAGS**

If you experience any of the following symptoms, do not proceed with your usual exercise routine or the exercises in this book. Always seek medical advice if you are unsure.

- **Any bleeding:** Spotting can be a normal symptom in early pregnancy, but it is worth getting checked just in case. Seek medical advice for a heavy bleed.
- **Sharp or stabbing abdominal pains:** You are bound to feel dull aches in the first trimester, but if they persist or become worse, seek advice from your midwife or GP before continuing with any exercise.
- **Any new aches and pains:** Within the back and pelvis and any associated change in sensation in your legs or feet. For a change in sensation around your bottom or genitals, seek urgent medical advice.
- **Signs of pelvic floor dysfunction:** These might be incontinence or prolapse symptoms, felt as a heavy dragging sensation in the vagina.

- **New wrist or hand pain:** Also numbness.
- **Shortness of breath.**
- **Dizziness:** Your blood pressure will usually be a little lower in early pregnancy, so dizziness can result from that. Sit down, drink plenty of water, and see if it eases. Do not exercise if you feel dizzy.
- **Excessive vomiting:** Nausea and vomiting are common pregnancy symptoms, but if you cannot keep anything down at all, not even fluids, then you should contact your GP or midwife and certainly not be exercising.

Conditions that are absolute contraindications to exercise: Uncontrolled type 1 diabetes, thyroid conditions and high blood pressure; concerns regarding the cervix; placenta praevia after 28 weeks; contractions that could be a sign of premature labour; signs of premature rupture of membranes (waters breaking).

EXERCISE IN THE
FIRST TRIMESTER

There is a lot of concern surrounding what is and isn't safe to do in early pregnancy, and understandably so. It is a whole new world and can feel very daunting. So, is it okay to exercise in the first trimester? Yes! This answer brings great relief to those women who enjoy exercise and use it as a means of staying on top of their mental as well as physical wellbeing. With pregnancy comes lots of new emotions, so it can be helpful to keep up some form of exercise for your mind. If you haven't already read them, see pages 8–9 for the overall safety guidelines before you start exercising.

I certainly enjoyed being able to stay active in the first 12 weeks, but even though it is a field I have worked in for over 10 years now, I still found myself feeling anxious about exercising at times. I noticed that my heart rate was higher than usual when exercising; on one occasion my Apple watch piped up and told me that I should consider stopping my workout when I was only in the warm-up. This proved to me that you need to listen to your body rather than get fixated on the numbers.

To assess the intensity of my workout, I would continually ask myself these four questions when exercising:

1. Can I breathe properly?
2. Could I talk if someone were to ask me a question now?
3. Am I at a comfortable temperature?
4. Is my heart rate coming down when I rest?

As long as you are answering yes to those four questions, you can rest assured that you are working at a sensible intensity for you. This is far better than trying to stick to a specific

WITH PREGNANCY COMES LOTS OF NEW EMOTIONS, SO IT CAN BE HELPFUL TO KEEP UP SOME FORM OF EXERCISE FOR YOUR MIND.

heart rate (we are all different, so there is no such thing as the 'ideal' heart rate zone) and your body will tell you quicker than anything or anyone else if you are pushing yourself too hard. If you are wearing a heart rate monitor, familiarize yourself with what range is good for your body and pull back a little when you notice it going too high for you.

NEW GOALS

You may find it difficult not being able to exercise at the level you could before. Remember, your goal is to be strong and fit for pregnancy, not to compete against your pre-pregnant self, win a race, hit a PB, or lose weight, and this can be a strange adjustment to make.

If you find it stressful to see the number on the scales going up, then bin them. I didn't weigh myself once in my pregnancy as I knew it wouldn't be good for my mental health. I did my best to eat a balanced diet (even when crisps were a large part of that!) and stay active, so I hoped that the majority of the weight I gained would be for the baby, but I just didn't need to see it on the scales. However, some pregnant women find it helpful to see the number on the scales

MISCARRIAGE CONCERNS

If you have previously miscarried, you may be concerned about exercising. After my second miscarriage I was petrified of doing anything to 'dislodge the baby', so in the next pregnancy I decided to stay as still as I could. When I miscarried again, as devastating as it was, it served as a reminder to me that it wasn't because of anything I'd 'done'. So, for this pregnancy I kept my exercise routine pretty much the same, but listened very closely to how my body was feeling each day. If I started to feel unwell, dizzy, or very out of breath at any stage, I took a break and lowered the intensity to a point where I felt okay again, or some days I just took it as a sign that I needed to rest. Your body is really busy during these first few weeks of pregnancy, so if it needs extra energy it will take it from you, leaving you little for yourself.

going up to remind them that their baby is growing, so do what feels best for you.

CARDIO EXERCISE

If you have the energy, you can still do cardio, unless your doctor has told you not to. If you find that your heart rate is slightly higher than usual, adjust your intensity and speed to make sure that you are working at a comfortable pace. If you're doing a class, it is important to tell the instructor that you are pregnant, even if you have to tell them on the sly. They can quietly give you variations and it will stop them picking on you if they think you're not making enough effort! Aim to work no harder than 70 per cent of your max – no more all-out sprints where you collapse on the floor from exhaustion!

I stopped running in the first few weeks of pregnancy as it didn't feel right for me. I am not a regular runner and I could feel a heavy pressure in my pelvis, so I made the decision to stick to low-impact cardio such as spinning and swimming instead. However, I know plenty of women who continue to enjoy running throughout their first trimester and further into their pregnancies.

STRENGTH TRAINING

Whether you are lifting weights or using your own body weight, working on your strength can benefit the body in so many ways during pregnancy.

There are old wives' tales about how pregnant women shouldn't stretch because their joint laxity increases, and whilst this second part is true it is still important to stretch. During pregnancy the levels of a hormone called relaxin increase, which has an effect on the soft tissues, leading to your muscles being able to stretch more. It's nothing to be concerned about, but be mindful of it and during stretches don't push into any pain. Go into stretches slowly and carefully and to a depth that feels right for you, but definitely still do them. Keeping your muscles strong through exercise helps to support joints during this process during pregnancy and beyond. Strength training doesn't have to mean lifting super-heavy weights – it is anything that helps you to build and maintain your strength. This can be Pilates-based workouts, bodyweight exercises, and workouts using resistance bands and weights – whatever you feel comfortable doing.

If you are new to exercise, then you can still start doing all of these things in pregnancy – just start slowly and ask for advice from a qualified trainer if and when you need it. Never be afraid to do so, as it is far better to ask than to do something anyway and then lose sleep over whether it was the right thing to do.

If you were used to lifting heavy weights pre-pregnancy, then there is nothing stopping you from continuing your weight training, but you must listen to your body. Now is not the time to be trying to beat your personal best or lift the heaviest weights. You should be aiming at around the 8-rep mark. If you can lift a weight without too much difficulty for 8–10 repetitions, then this is a sensible intensity to be working at. Remember that you are aiming for

IF YOU WERE USED TO LIFTING HEAVY WEIGHTS PRE-PREGNANCY, THERE IS NOTHING STOPPING YOU FROM CONTINUING YOUR WEIGHT TRAINING, BUT YOU MUST LISTEN TO YOUR BODY.

70 per cent max for all types of training, not just cardio.

It is important to keep your whole body strong during pregnancy, but there are some specific areas it is useful to focus on:

- Your glutes need to be switched on and active in order to support the changes that will come in the pelvis and your posture; your lower back will thank you too.
- As your posture changes, it is easy to round your shoulders and hunch your upper back, so keeping those muscles strong will help you to stand up straight and avoid getting an achy neck and back.

• The core needs to stay strong to help support your bump, but how you strengthen it is different in pregnancy.

A STRONG CORE

You can do lots to keep your core strong, but you have to adapt the exercises. Gone are the days when you work your abs so hard you can't laugh without feeling them for a week afterwards! For now you have to be kind to your core and look after it as it houses your baby.

In the first trimester, you may not have a bump and until it starts to appear you can continue with your usual core exercises. However, it is worth starting to prepare and get into good habits for when your bump begins to show. I started adapting my exercises pretty early on and I am glad that I did. My core felt super-strong and supportive until the end of my pregnancy. Just because you aren't smashing out the sit-ups does not mean that your core can't be strong.

It is incredibly important to get into good breathing habits early on to learn to engage your core without thinking too much about it. The core muscles we want to focus on throughout pregnancy are the deep ones that you can't necessarily see – the transverse abdominis (often known as the TVA). When you exhale, you are able to gently engage these muscles and use them to help stabilize your body whilst doing an exercise, as well as maintain their strength as your bump grows.

REST DAYS

I am a big believer in scheduling in rest days to allow your body to recover, but even more so in pregnancy. Your body is doing so much that you can't see, and trust me when I say that you will soon look forward to those rest days more than ever before. It is very common to feel exhausted in the first trimester and totally understandable given the amount of changes going on in your body. It is important to know when to give in to that exhaustion and give your body the rest that it needs.

There is a difference between feeling tired at the end of a long day and the total and utter exhaustion that can come over you in pregnancy. I remember feeling that if I didn't have a nap immediately, I might fall asleep standing up. I have never been someone who naps, but I would wake up in the morning and turn straight to my diary to see where I could schedule one in that afternoon between clients. I just knew I would need it.

To avoid falling asleep standing up or at your desk, especially if you are still keeping your pregnancy a secret at work, try to stay ahead of the game and make sure you are getting enough rest. This might mean going to bed early, not

ENGAGING **YOUR CORE**

Adding in a new breathing technique to your exercise routine can be tricky, but if you practise and perfect it in your first trimester it will become second nature to you later on. An easy way to remember it is with the three Es:

Exhale and Engage on the Exertion

Here's how to do it: Just before you start performing the hardest part of any exercise, such as standing back up in the squat or coming up in your press-up, begin to breathe out and gently engage your deep core muscles by hugging your baby in towards your spine. This way you are making sure that these muscles are fully switched on and helping you perform the exercise. Try to look at all exercises as core exercises in one way or another, because by using your breath effectively you can bring the core into almost every movement that you do.

If this is not your first pregnancy or your bump has made a nice early appearance, you'll need to start adapting your core exercises as per the second trimester. Head to page 110 to read more.

exercising on back-to-back days, or lowering the number of cardio sessions you do each week. Whatever you can do to stay on top of your energy levels will be super-helpful.

PELVIC FLOOR EXERCISES

It is never too soon to start pelvic floor exercises during pregnancy, and you should aim to strengthen your pelvic floor whether you are pregnant or not.

The muscles sit at the base of the pelvis and have some very important jobs, including maintaining continence of urine, faeces, and wind; supporting your pelvic organs during pregnancy; contributing to sexual pleasure; working with other core muscles to support the spine; and moving lymph fluid and blood around the area.

We talk about exercising the pelvic floor muscles so much in pregnancy because the process of carrying a baby weakens and lengthens them. Therefore, we need to work on strengthening them to counteract this process. Research has shown that doing pelvic floor exercises in early pregnancy reduces the risk of developing incontinence towards the end of pregnancy or after birth.

To engage the pelvic floor correctly, imagine holding in wind or squeeze your

> IT IS NEVER TOO SOON TO START PELVIC FLOOR EXERCISES DURING PREGNANCY – AIM TO DO THEM WHETHER YOU ARE PREGNANT OR NOT.

anus. However, some women find other cues better or easier to follow, such as imagining closing a zip from the back passage to front passage, or imagining stopping the flow of urine mid-flow. Letting go of the muscles is as important as the squeeze. We want strong and flexible pelvic floor muscles.

- **Short exercise:** Contract (squeeze) and let go, so hold wind (squeeze your anus) and let go. Aim for 10 of these, ensuring you are letting go between each one.

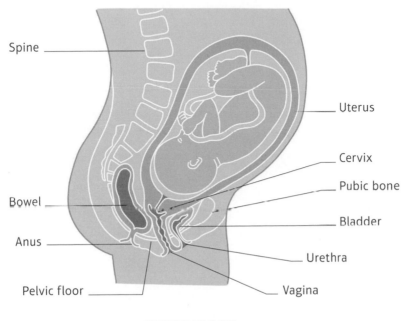

Spine

Uterus

Cervix

Pubic bone

Bowel

Bladder

Anus

Urethra

Pelvic floor

Vagina

PELVIC FLOOR

- **Long exercise:** Contract and hold for 10 seconds, while breathing in and out gently, then let go. Do not hold your breath or worry if 10 seconds is not possible at the beginning. The advice is to try 10 of each, three times a day. Slowly build them into your routine.

A few top pelvic floor tips are:

- Relax your tummy, legs, and bottom muscles.
- Try to do at least one set while standing. Do as many standing as possible.

- Keep the muscles relaxed as you breathe in and contract them as you breathe out. The diaphragm sits above the pelvic floor and they work together.
- Download the NHS Squeezy app, which has advice and reminders.
- See a pelvic health physiotherapist (see page 203) if you are struggling with the exercises, are incontinent, or are experiencing other symptoms such as prolapse, which may present as a heavy or dragging feeling within the vagina.

FIRST TRIMESTER
WORKOUT PLAN

The workouts in this section are suitable for the first trimester, but if the number of repetitions seems a bit high for you, or even a bit low, feel free to adapt them to the level that feels right for you. You may notice that your heart rate increases a little more than you are used to during pregnancy, but that is completely normal – just take rest breaks when you need them and keep hydrated before, during, and after your workout. There are 12 workouts for you to try – a mix of upper body, lower body, and full body. For instructions on how to do each exercise, see the Pose Directory on pages 36–61 and look out for the modification notes next to some of the exercises. You can spread the workouts out evenly with three each week, or if you prefer to repeat one workout you particularly like a few times, then that is fine. The workouts are there to guide you, but choose what feels right for you and mix it up a little if you want to. Always listen to your body and don't forget to do the warm-up and cool-down exercises (see pages 26–33).

UPPER BODY
WORKOUT 1

CIRCUIT A

1. Alternating shoulder press x20 (p48)

2. Tricep extension x15 (p54)

3. Plank march x10 (p48)

4. Renegade row x10 alternating (p51)

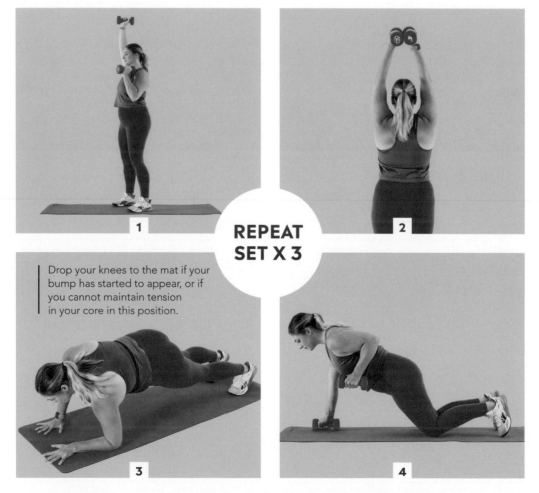

1

REPEAT SET X 3

2

Drop your knees to the mat if your bump has started to appear, or if you cannot maintain tension in your core in this position.

3

4

CIRCUIT B

1. Curl & press x15 (p50)

2. Press-up x10 (p46)

3. Wide shoulder press x10 (p49)

4. Arm raise x10 alternating (p47)

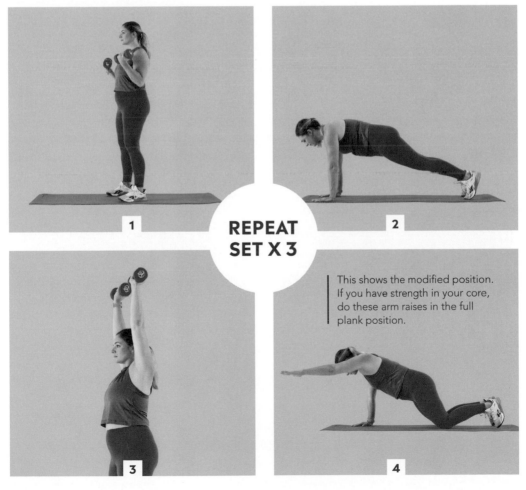

REPEAT SET X 3

This shows the modified position. If you have strength in your core, do these arm raises in the full plank position.

UPPER BODY
WORKOUT 2

CIRCUIT A

1. Alternating shoulder press x15 (p48)

2. Bentover row x15 (p50)

3. Curl & press x15 (p50)

4. Plank march x10 (p48)

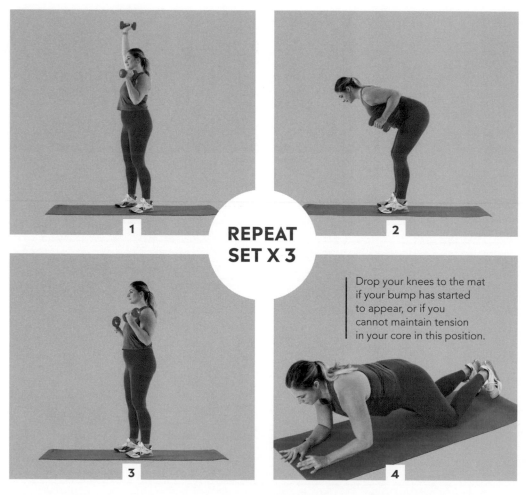

REPEAT SET X 3

Drop your knees to the mat if your bump has started to appear, or if you cannot maintain tension in your core in this position.

CIRCUIT B

1. Frontal raise x10 (p53)

2. Chest press x15 (p55)

3. Side plank twist x10 each side (p58)

4. Shoulder tap x10 alternating (p60)

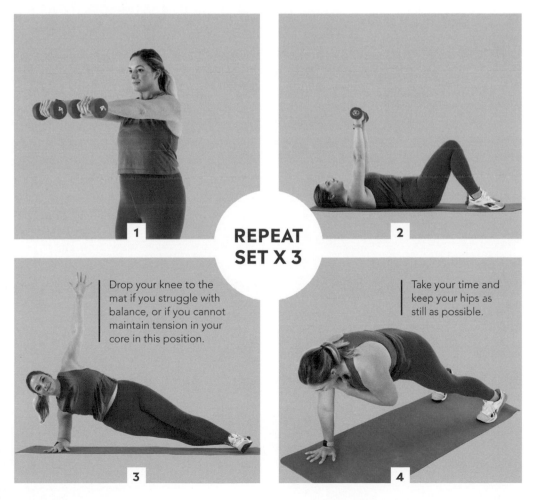

REPEAT SET X 3

Drop your knee to the mat if you struggle with balance, or if you cannot maintain tension in your core in this position.

Take your time and keep your hips as still as possible.

UPPER BODY
WORKOUT 3

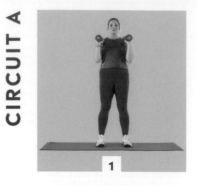

CIRCUIT A

1. Narrow shoulder press x15 (p49)

2. Bentover row x10 (p50)

3. Press-up x1 and 1 tap each shoulder x10 (p47)

4. Chest flyes x15 (p57)

REPEAT SET X 3

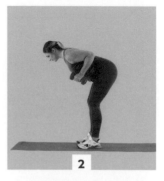

CIRCUIT B

1. Alternating shoulder press x20 (p48)

2. Lateral raise x10 (p53)

3. Plank march x10 (p48)

4. Arm raise x10 alternating (p47)

REPEAT SET X 3

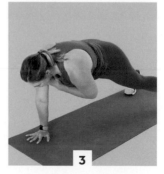

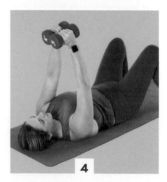

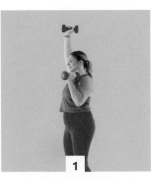

1

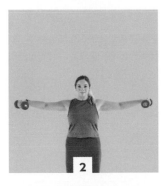

2

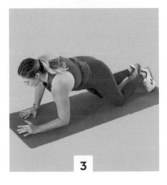

3

Drop your knees to the mat if your bump has started to appear, or if you cannot maintain tension in your core in a full plank.

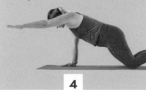

4

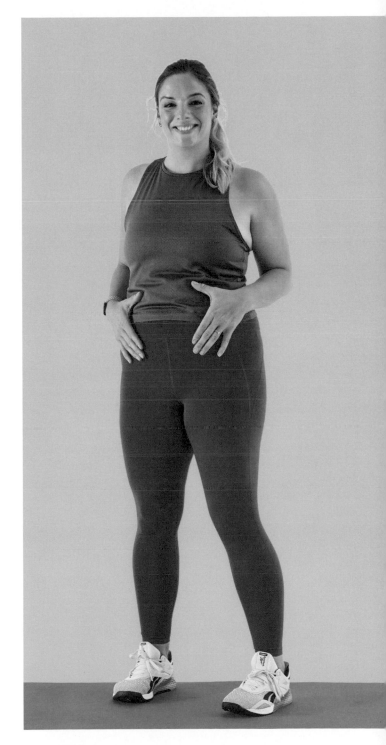

UPPER BODY
WORKOUT 4

CIRCUIT A

1. Press-up x10 (p46)

2. Wide shoulder press x10 (p49)

3. Renegade row x10 alternating (p51)

4. Side plank crunch x10 each side (p59)

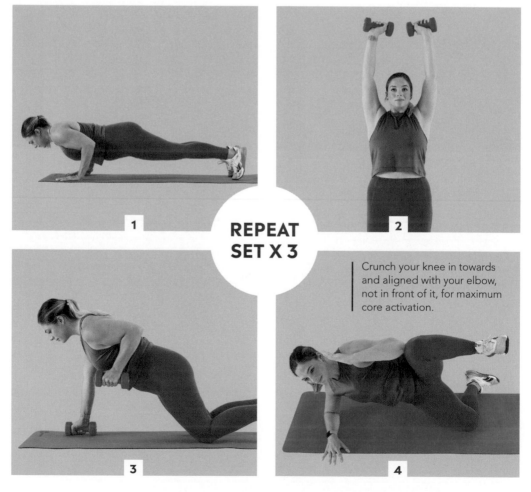

REPEAT SET X 3

Crunch your knee in towards and aligned with your elbow, not in front of it, for maximum core activation.

CIRCUIT B

1. Tricep extension x15 (p54)

2. Single bentover row x10 each side (p51)

3. Chest press x10 (p55)

4. Chest flyes x10 (p57)

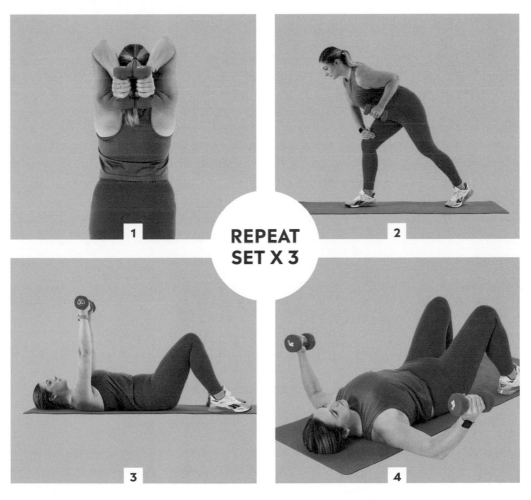

REPEAT SET X 3

LOWER BODY
WORKOUT 5

CIRCUIT A

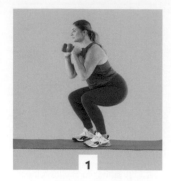

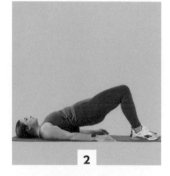

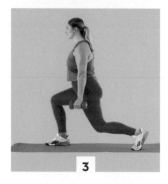

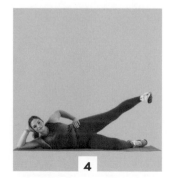

CIRCUIT A

1. Pulsing squat 3 pulses x10 (p36)

2. Glute bridge x10 (p43)

3. Backward lunge x20 alternating (p38)

4. Lying leg raise x10 each side (p44)

CIRCUIT B

1. Bodyweight squat x10 (p36)

2. Side lunge x10 alternating (p40)

3. Lying leg crunch x10 each side (p45)

4. Side plank twist x10 each side (p58)

REPEAT SET X 3

CIRCUIT B

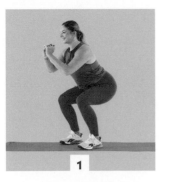

1

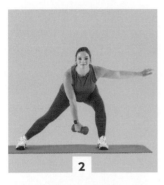

2

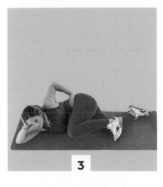

3

Drop your knee to the mat if you struggle with balance, or if you cannot maintain tension in your core in this position.

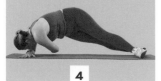

4

REPEAT SET X 3

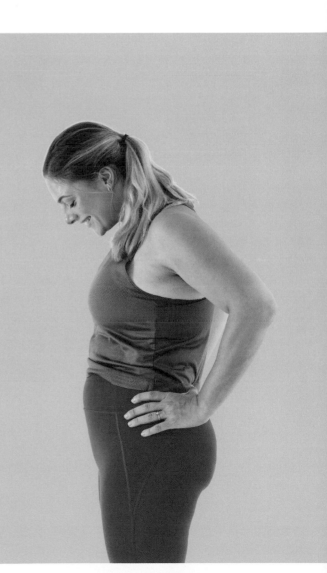

LOWER BODY
WORKOUT 6

CIRCUIT A

1. Sumo deadlift x15 (p42)

2. Side lunge x10 alternating (p40)

3. Single glute bridge x10 each side (p43)

4. Bird dog x10 each side (p60)

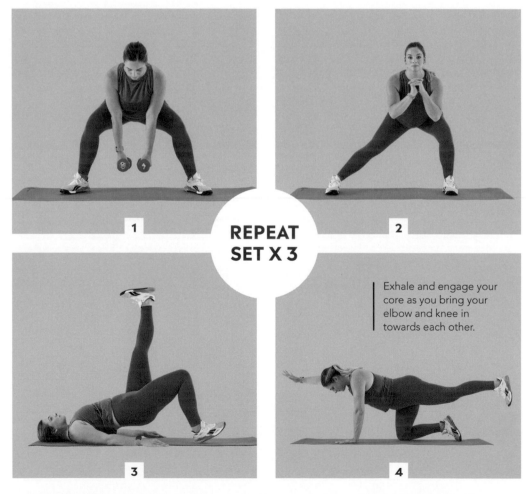

REPEAT SET X 3

Exhale and engage your core as you bring your elbow and knee in towards each other.

CIRCUIT B

1. Balance lunge x10 each side (p38)

2. Pulsing squat 3 pulses x10 (p36)

3. Lying leg raise x10 each side (p44)

4. 4-point knee raise x5–10 (p61)

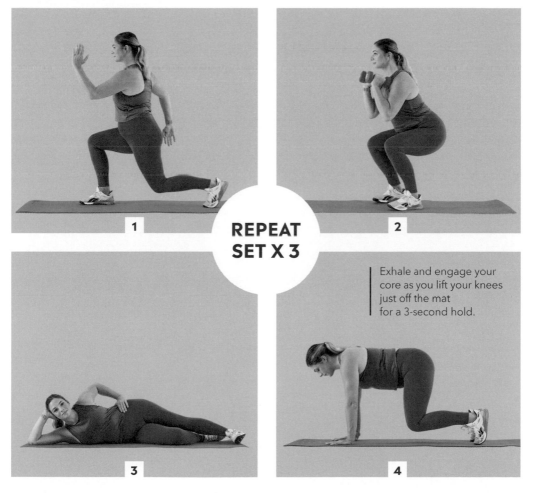

REPEAT SET X 3

1

2

Exhale and engage your core as you lift your knees just off the mat for a 3-second hold.

3

4

LOWER BODY
WORKOUT 7

CIRCUIT A

1. Romanian Deadlift (RDL) x10 (p41)

2. Balance lunge x10 each side (p38)

3. Glute bridge x15 (p43)

4. Side plank dip x10 each side (p59)

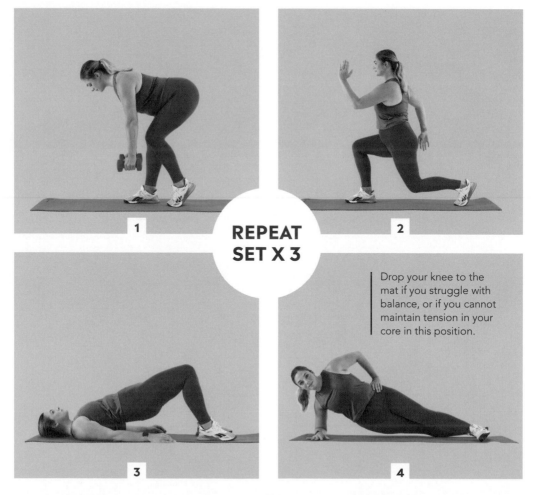

REPEAT SET X 3

Drop your knee to the mat if you struggle with balance, or if you cannot maintain tension in your core in this position.

CIRCUIT B

1. Sumo squat x15 (p37)

2. Static lunge x10 each side (p39)

3. Lying leg raise x 10 each side (p44)

4. Lying leg crunch x10 each side (p45)

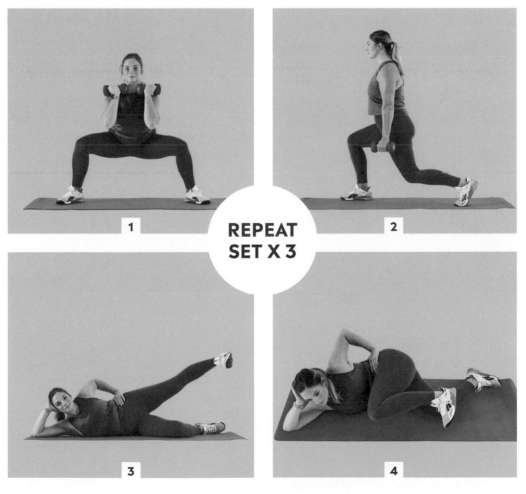

REPEAT
SET X 3

LOWER BODY
WORKOUT 8

CIRCUIT A

1. Pulsing squat 3 pulses x10 (p36)

2. Side lunge x10 alternating (p40)

3. Modified burpee x10 (p45)

4. Glute bridge x15 (p43)

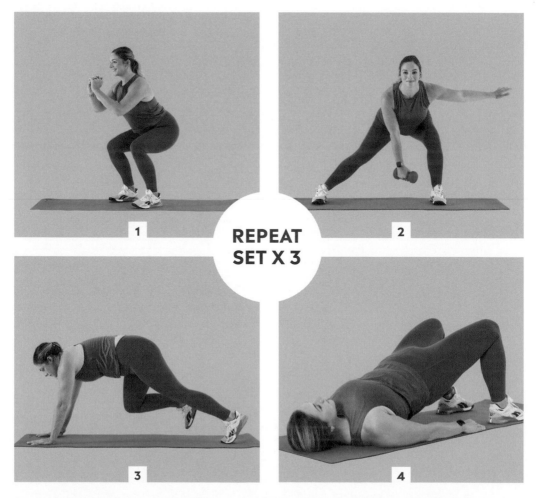

REPEAT SET X 3

CIRCUIT B

1. Romanian Deadlift (RDL) x15 (p41)

2. Bird dog x10 each side (p60)

3. Single RDL x10 each side (p42)

4. Side plank dip x10 each side (p59)

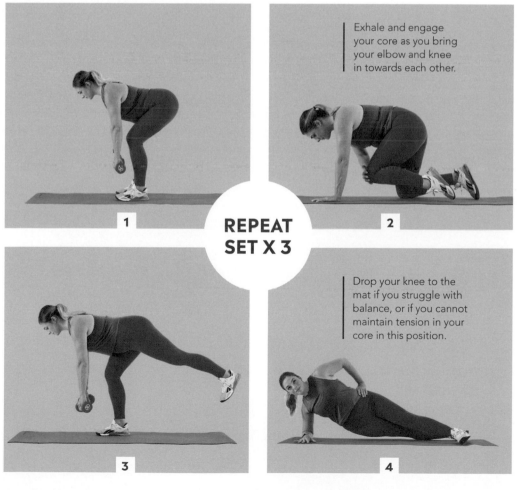

Exhale and engage your core as you bring your elbow and knee in towards each other.

1

REPEAT SET X 3

2

Drop your knee to the mat if you struggle with balance, or if you cannot maintain tension in your core in this position.

3

4

FULL BODY
WORKOUT 9

CIRCUIT A

1. Squat & press x10 (p37)

2. Glute bridge chest press x15 (p56)

3. Single bentover row x10 each side (p51)

4. Side plank crunch x10 each side (p59)

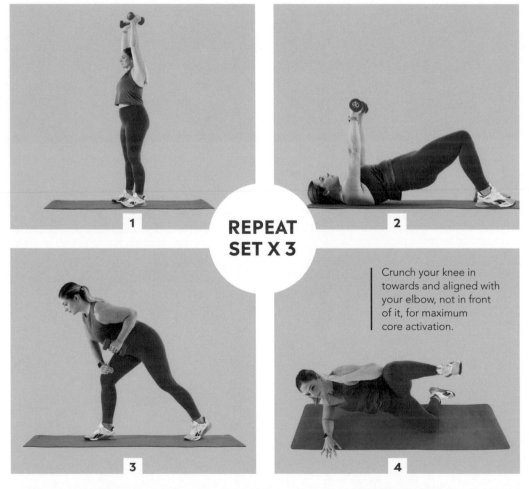

REPEAT SET X 3

Crunch your knee in towards and aligned with your elbow, not in front of it, for maximum core activation.

CIRCUIT B

1. Modified burpee x10 (p45)

2. Lunge & curl x20 alternating (p39)

3. Renegade row x10 alternating (p51)

4. Shoulder tap x20 alternating (p60)

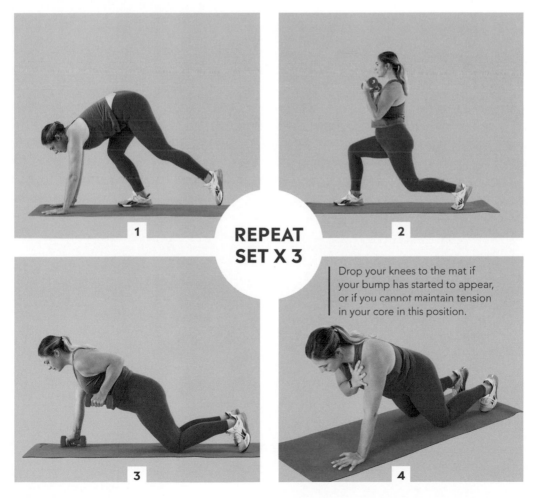

REPEAT SET X 3

Drop your knees to the mat if your bump has started to appear, or if you cannot maintain tension in your core in this position.

FULL BODY
WORKOUT 10

CIRCUIT A

1. Side lunge x10 alternating (p40)

2. Frontal & lateral raise x10 (p53)

3. Modified burpee x10 (p45)

4. Chest press x15 (p55)

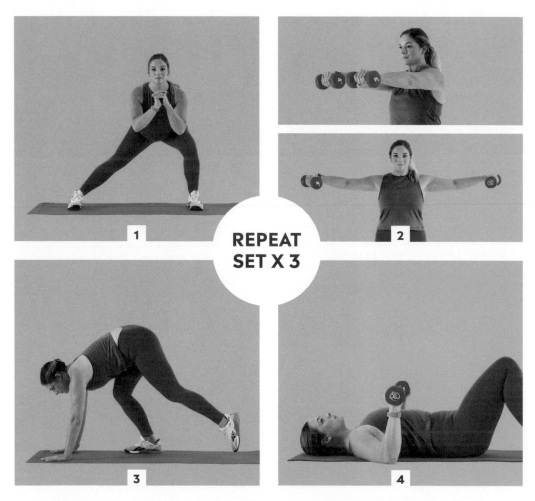

REPEAT SET X 3

CIRCUIT B

1. Pulsing squat 3 pulses x15 (p36)

2. Renegade row x10 alternating (p51)

3. Backward lunge x20 alternating (p38)

4. Bird dog x10 each side (p60)

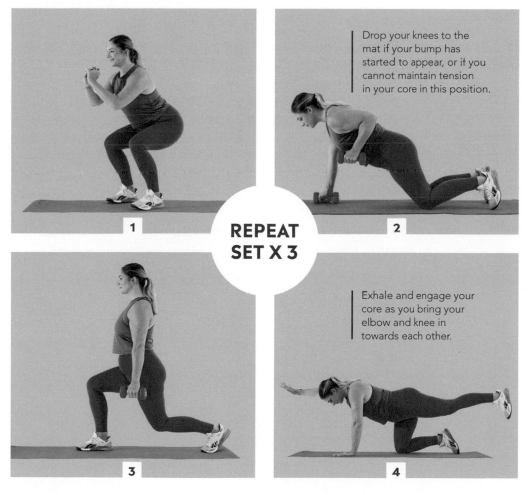

Drop your knees to the mat if your bump has started to appear, or if you cannot maintain tension in your core in this position.

REPEAT
SET X 3

Exhale and engage your core as you bring your elbow and knee in towards each other.

FULL BODY
WORKOUT 11

CIRCUIT A

1. Pulsing squat 3 pulses x15 (p36)

2. Tricep extension x15 (p54)

3. Single glute bridge x10 each side (p43)

4. Side plank twist x10 each side (p58)

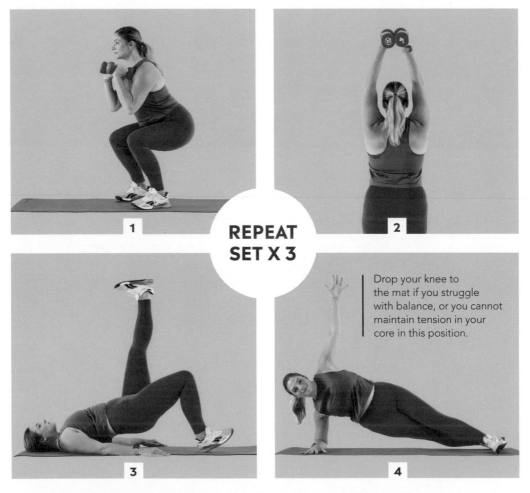

REPEAT SET X 3

Drop your knee to the mat if you struggle with balance, or you cannot maintain tension in your core in this position.

CIRCUIT B

1. Balance lunge x10 each side (p38)

2. Upright row x10 (p52)

3. Glute bridge chest press x15 (p56)

4. 4-point knee raise x5–10 (p61)

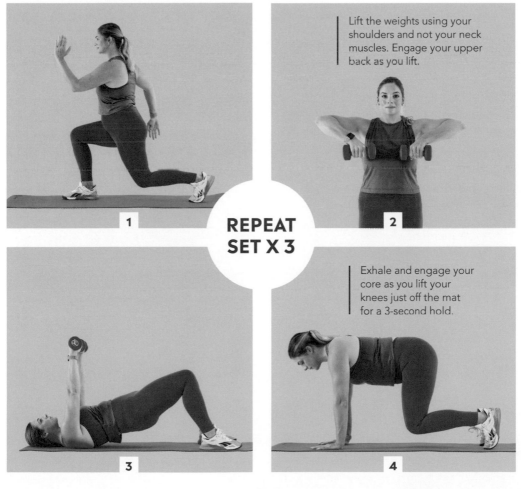

Lift the weights using your shoulders and not your neck muscles. Engage your upper back as you lift.

REPEAT SET X 3

Exhale and engage your core as you lift your knees just off the mat for a 3-second hold.

FULL BODY
WORKOUT 12

CIRCUIT A

1. Squat & press x10 (p37)

2. Press-up x1 and 1 tap each shoulder x10 (p47)

3. Sumo squat x10 (p37)

4. Upright row x10 (p52)

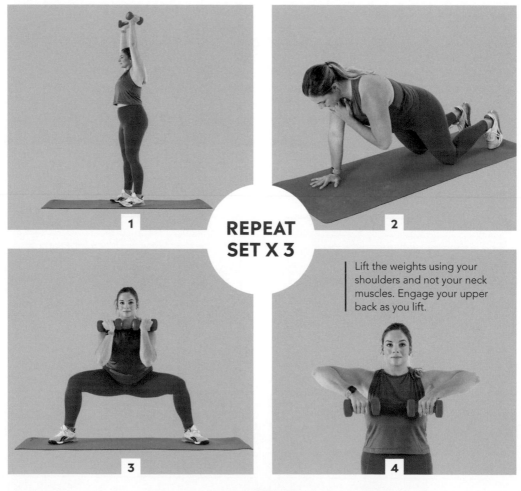

REPEAT SET X 3

Lift the weights using your shoulders and not your neck muscles. Engage your upper back as you lift.

CIRCUIT B

1. Frontal & lateral raise x10 (p53)

2. Side lunge x10 alternating (p40)

3. Narrow shoulder press x10 (p49)

4. Shoulder tap x10–20 alternating (p60)

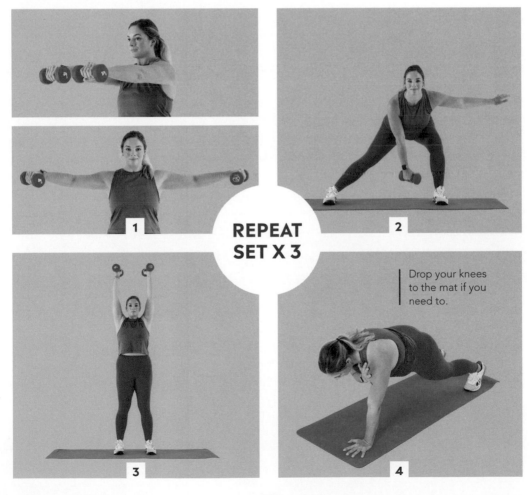

REPEAT SET X 3

Drop your knees to the mat if you need to.

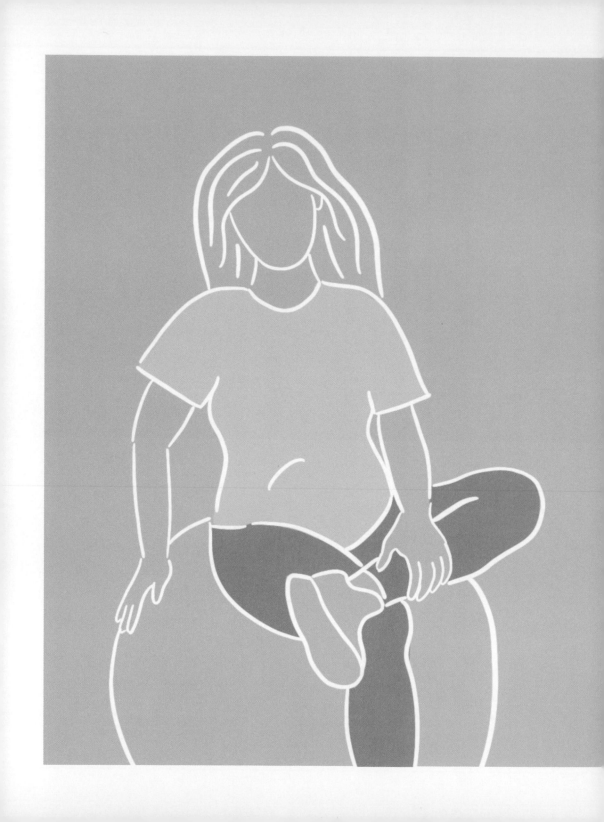

SECOND TRIMESTER
Weeks 13–27

The pregnancy 'glow' doesn't happen for all women, but hopefully you will have more energy and fewer symptoms to deal with during this middle trimester. As your bump gets bigger, hiding your pregnancy will be a thing of the past!

WHAT TO EXPECT IN
THE SECOND TRIMESTER

The second trimester of pregnancy is from 13–27 weeks. This is often a big milestone and when people tend to start telling their family and friends the good news, if they haven't already. It couldn't come soon enough for me. I was petrified, constantly worrying about the 'what ifs', still Googling ridiculous things, and just hoping with every ounce of me that we would come away from our 12-week scan with happy news.

We did! Again there must have been a warning sign on my file saying "very anxious" because there was no dilly-dallying and with a bit of cold jelly on my tummy, we could soon see a very wriggly baby. The sonographer's smile was almost as big as ours. George squeezed my hand the entire time – we just couldn't believe how much the baby had grown since the last scan and how active it was. It seemed to be doing a little workout! I wonder where it inherited that from?

The scan took a little longer than usual, as it was tricky to get all the measurements, but I didn't mind. The longer I could see my amazing baby on the screen, the better. Everything looked fine and I couldn't sense any doubt in the sonographer's tone. We asked lots of questions and were soon on our way out of the hospital feeling happier than we could ever imagine being. I couldn't believe I was finally getting that string of black-and-white baby pictures that I had seen so many other people come away with over the years. It was finally our turn. We were on top of the world, and into our second trimester!

FEELING BETTER?

So this is the magical second trimester where everything is meant to feel great and all those nasty symptoms supposedly disappear, right? Maybe, but not always. Some poor women draw all the short straws in pregnancy and may even have morning sickness for the entirety, but hopefully you are not one of them

Whatever your pregnancy symptoms, and however long they last, try not to compare them to anyone else's. If you

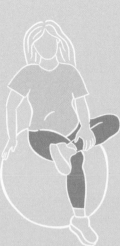

YOUR BABY **IN THE SECOND TRIMESTER**

For many women, this is the most comfortable and enjoyable trimester. Your baby has been very busy growing over the last few weeks, and can yawn, hiccup, swallow, and even taste the things you eat through the amniotic fluid, but don't worry, they won't come out with an in-built love for chocolate biscuits, or crisps in my case!

Your baby's senses are developing so they can now hear your voice as well as your partner's voice, so talk to them lots and play nice music to your bump. The other senses, such as smell and sight, are developing too. Towards the latter weeks of this trimester, try shining a light on your bump, or clapping loudly over it to see if it makes your baby move. We sometimes found this worked for us.

Your baby will start to pack on the pounds from about week 23 and by the end of your first trimester will weigh around 1kg (2lb).

feel absolutely awful and see no signs of it easing up, speak to your GP as there are things they can prescribe to help. Be reassured that it doesn't mean there is anything wrong with you or your baby – every woman is different.

I didn't get that magical surge of energy at 12 weeks – in fact, I felt pretty exhausted still. I spent the first few weeks of the second trimester wondering if I was ever going to feel better and have more energy again. Thankfully, towards

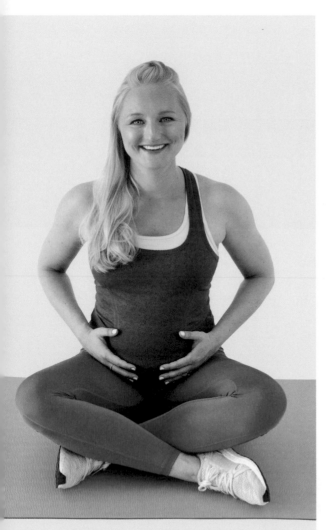

the 20-week mark I started to feel more myself and I was extremely grateful. My energy started to return and I felt more motivated to exercise and start socializing again.

YOUR BUMP

If this is your first pregnancy, the likelihood is that your bump will take a little while to show, but that's certainly not the case for everyone. While I was kept waiting until around 18 weeks to be able to see anything significant, some of my friends started showing at around 10 weeks. As with everything in pregnancy, it is unhelpful to make comparisons but it is also so difficult not to, especially in your first pregnancy when everything is new.

When your bump starts to show, it launches you into that awkward phase of people wondering whether you are pregnant or whether you've just had a big lunch! So that was when I wore baggy jumpers all the time. Perhaps this is why women often decide to wear a baby on board badge early on, to avoid any uncertainty, but I just decided to wear loose and comfortable clothes until the bump made an appearance.

FEELING THE BABY KICK

Some women feel the baby kick for the first time from about 16 weeks, but it can happen weeks later than this, especially if it is your first pregnancy. I was told at my 12-week scan that my placenta was anterior, meaning it was in front of my baby. Though this wouldn't have a negative impact on the pregnancy, it meant it might take me longer to feel any movement. Great, as if I wasn't anxious enough – now I had to wait even longer to feel those reassuring kicks! It didn't stop me keeping a very close eye out for anything that might resemble a kick… or was it wind? Hard to tell in pregnancy really, isn't it?

At around 18 weeks I felt one or two tiny movements, which were like popcorn popping in a microwave, but they were not distinct and would only happen once every few days. Everyone told me it would feel like a flutter, but mine didn't.

On the day I turned 20 weeks, I was sitting in my car and suddenly felt something that was quite clearly a kick – it made me jump. I started giggling to myself, out of happiness and just pure relief, I think.

Those kicks were a huge milestone for me and I felt less anxious because I was getting regular reassurance that my baby was moving around. Of course, the next challenge was getting George to feel the kicks. I'd yell out to him every time I thought there might be one coming, only for the baby to stop at that exact moment. This went on for a week or so until one night George lay his head on my tummy and sure enough the baby kicked him directly in the head! He definitely felt that! From then on, every night before we went to sleep, he would lie with his hands on my tummy talking to the baby and feeling out for those kicks, which very quickly became stronger and more regular. It was like our goodnight to the baby, although of course I would go on to hear from it over and over again throughout the night during its 3am dance parties! That was fun!

EXERCISE IN THE
SECOND TRIMESTER

If you have renewed energy, then you may be excited to get back to a more regular exercise routine in the second trimester, but be mindful not to overdo it. If anyone, pregnant or not, took near enough 12 weeks off exercise, I wouldn't be sending them back in at the deep end. I would be advising them to ease back in and be kind to themselves. If you have managed to keep your exercise up in the first trimester, then continue with as much as you feel you can.

ADAPTING EXERCISE

Using weights is fine, and encouraged, as long as you are working with a weight and intensity that feels comfortable. Your body has changed over the last few weeks, so give yourself time to adapt before tackling weights or start with lighter ones than you used before. Your bump will now be dictating most of the adaptations you'll need to make throughout the second trimester, and as it starts to grow, you will want to alter your posture to make way for it. You might want to change the set-up of your bike in spinning to allow some more room for your tummy, or stand with your legs a little wider in a squat or deadlift for the same reason.

Lying flat on your back for long periods of time is not recommended at this stage of pregnancy as the entire weight of your uterus and baby can press down on the vena cava – a major vein that takes blood back to your heart from your lower body. Don't panic, though – you will feel breathless or even a little nauseous before anything worrying even begins to happen, so this is your sign to move positions. You can do this by elevating the top of the bench

YOUR POSTURE WILL BE AFFECTED AS YOUR BABY GROWS AND YOUR CENTRE OF GRAVITY MOVES FORWARDS. EXERCISE REALLY HELPS YOUR BODY AS IT ADAPTS TO THIS CHANGE IN POSTURE.

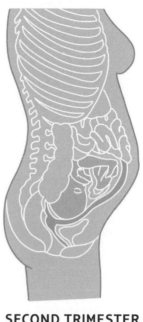

you're using, or leaning back against a sofa or a big cushion if you're at home, to keep you a little more upright. Don't be afraid to be on your back for short periods of time getting from one position to the next; the advice is just not to stay there for a long time. Tune in to how you feel and if you start to feel unwell or short of breath, then you know to move.

Your posture will be affected as your baby grows and your centre of gravity moves forwards. Exercise really helps your body as it adapts to this change in posture. It is common for the pelvis to tilt slightly forwards and for the curves of the back to increase. The increased size of your breasts also has an impact on your back – making sure you are wearing the right size bra is important for breast health and also your neck and back. You may experience discomfort in your back, or an increased feeling of stiffness.

CARDIO EXERCISE

As in the first trimester, the type of cardio exercise you do will largely depend on how you feel. As long as you are

SECOND TRIMESTER

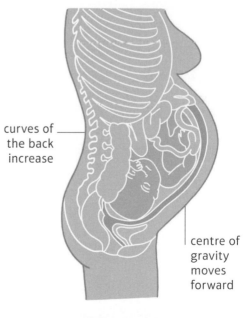

curves of the back increase

centre of gravity moves forward

THIRD TRIMESTER

managing the intensity of your workout and your heart rate stays at a comfortable pace, then you are okay to continue. As your bump gets bigger, you will find that you need to adapt as things begin to feel harder. Don't be disheartened – it makes sense that your body will have to work harder to keep up.

> AS YOUR BUMP GETS BIGGER, IT MAKES SENSE THAT YOUR BODY WILL HAVE TO WORK HARDER TO KEEP UP.

Often women stop running towards the end of this trimester, but if you are a seasoned runner, you may feel that your body is still coping well. Just make sure that you are constantly checking in with yourself and don't ignore any niggles.

STRENGTH TRAINING

The importance of strength grows as your pregnancy progresses, especially if you are keeping some form of impact in your exercise routine. Whether you are using heavy weights, light weights, or no weights at all, keep up with your strength training and you will find that the changes in posture will not bother you as much as they could – your body will be strong enough to cope with them. Remember, also, that upper body strength will stand you in good stead for all that lifting and carrying once your little one arrives.

Stick to the 8–10 repetitions rule, no matter how used you are to lifting weights. If you can't get to 8–10 repetitions of an exercise without a big struggle, consider using lighter weights and build up gradually.

PROTECTING YOUR CORE

Now you are in the second trimester, it is important to adapt exercises in order to protect your core, as your abdominal wall begins to stretch with your growing baby. It is perfectly normal for your core muscles to stretch apart (see opposite), otherwise the baby wouldn't be able to fit in your tummy, so don't worry – it doesn't hurt nor are you likely to feel the muscles stretching, but you do need to be mindful about the way in which you exercise to protect your core.

Diastasis

The abdominal muscles are designed with a gap down the middle, joined by a connective tissue called the linea alba. The linea alba needs to stretch so there is room for your baby to grow, which makes perfect sense. Diastasis Rectus Abdominus is the scientific term given to the thinning and widening of that connective tissue, which joins your six-pack muscles (rectus abdominal muscles), and yes you do have them whether you can see them or not!

Research has shown that all pregnant women will have some degree of diastasis by 35 weeks, so it isn't anything

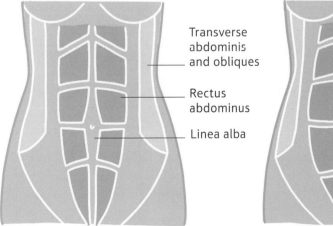

Transverse abdominis and obliques

Rectus abdominus

Linea alba

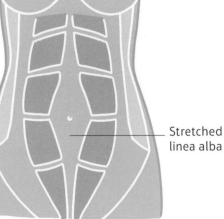

Stretched linea alba

NORMAL ABDOMEN

DIASTASIS

you've done wrong. The very thought of the abdominals stretching apart can cause anxiety and stress to some pregnant women, and the word diastasis

IT IS PERFECTLY NORMAL FOR YOUR CORE MUSCLES TO STRETCH APART, OTHERWISE THE BABY WOULDN'T BE ABLE TO FIT IN YOUR TUMMY.

is so often thrown around as a scaremongering tool.

There isn't a definitive list of risk factors that cause diastasis, but some considered to play a part are genetics, multiple pregnancies, and having a shorter torso. Some women will start pregnancy with a slightly larger gap between their muscles.

As you exercise, you may notice a coning or doming shape down the centre of your tummy, especially during sit-ups, crunches, double leg raises, full plank

holds, or any exercise done in a full plank position. These are not the only exercises where you might see doming – there isn't an exact list of dos and don'ts or when to stop each exercise, as everyone is different, but understanding what to look for and when to modify is the key.

If you see your tummy creating a cone shape, it is simply a sign that whatever movement you are doing is too much for your core to handle right now so it needs modifying, but that doesn't mean you can't work your core at all.

Engaging the core

There are ways to adapt traditional core exercises, which you will see in the second trimester workouts in this section, but there are also plenty of ways to make sure the core is engaged whilst doing upper and lower body exercises too, and that is through using your breath.

Ensuring you do deep diaphragmatic breathing and know how to engage and use the deep abdominal muscles is important to help your tummy during pregnancy. Remember your three Es (see page 75).

You might also notice the doming during everyday activities, such as getting out of bed, hoisting yourself off the sofa, getting out of the bath; all these movements can involve increased pressure within the tummy. Get into the habit of turning yourself on to your side or on to all-fours and continue this in the postnatal period. It's not very ladylike, but it will help a great deal.

Another activity that can put a lot of pressure through the tummy is going for a poo, made worse if you are constipated and straining. Making sure you drink enough water, have enough fibre in your diet, sit on the toilet with your feet raised, maybe supported on a little step, and taking deep breaths can really help. If you are struggling with constipation, speak to your GP or midwife for advice.

USING **A GYM**

While the workouts in this book are designed to be done anywhere, you may have access to a gym and want to use some of the equipment there as well.

Of course, there is nothing stopping you from exercising in a gym when you are pregnant, but if you are unsure of how to use any of the equipment, or feel unwell at any point, get help from one of the personal trainers or another member of staff.

Cross trainers, stationary bikes, and treadmills are all safe to use during pregnancy, but always be mindful of your set-up, and to avoid falling, never go faster than feels comfortable. Remember to only work to 70 per cent maximum effort.

The same goes for any exercise classes you might want to attend; always go at your own pace and make it known to the instructor that you are pregnant.

SECOND TRIMESTER
WORKOUT PLAN

I'm crossing everything that you have got some energy back after a tiring first trimester. If you haven't yet, don't worry – you may gradually find more energy in the coming weeks. In this section there's another set of 12 workouts. See the Pose Directory on pages 36–61 for how to do each exercise and look out for the modification notes next to some of the exercises. Don't forget to do the warm-up and cool-down exercises (see pages 26–33). You'll notice that some of the exercises have been adapted slightly to make allowances for your bump as it starts to appear, but hopefully they are all exercises that you are now familiar with if you've been doing them during the first trimester. Use the repetition ranges as a guide only – do less if you need to or more if you feel that you can. Always listen to your body. Drink plenty of water and take rest breaks as and when you need them. Your body will be carrying some extra weight now, so don't be surprised if things start to feel a little harder than they used to.

UPPER BODY
WORKOUT 1

CIRCUIT A

1. Renegade row x10 alternating (p51)

2. Press-up x10 (p46)

3. Narrow shoulder press x10 (p49)

4. Tricep dip x10 (p54)

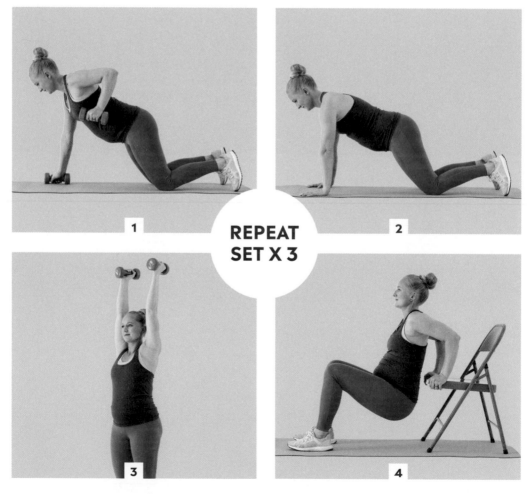

REPEAT SET X 3

CIRCUIT B

1. Wide shoulder press x10 (p49)

2. Bicep curl x10 (p52)

3. Reverse table top dip x10 (p46)

4. Belly breathing x5 rounds (p61)

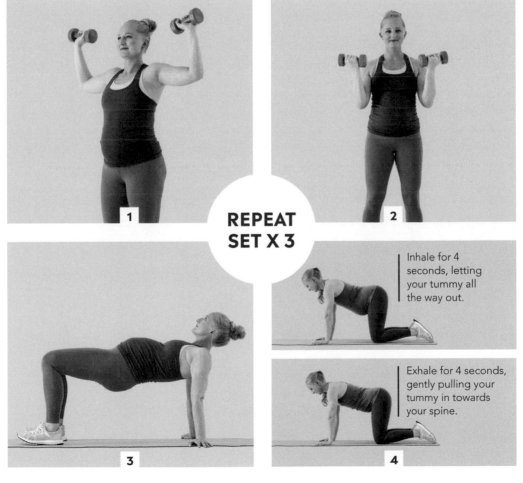

REPEAT SET X 3

Inhale for 4 seconds, letting your tummy all the way out.

Exhale for 4 seconds, gently pulling your tummy in towards your spine.

UPPER BODY
WORKOUT 2

CIRCUIT A

1. Curl & press x10 (p50)

2. Single bentover row x10 (p51)

3. Press-up x10 (p46)

4. Lateral raise x10 (p53)

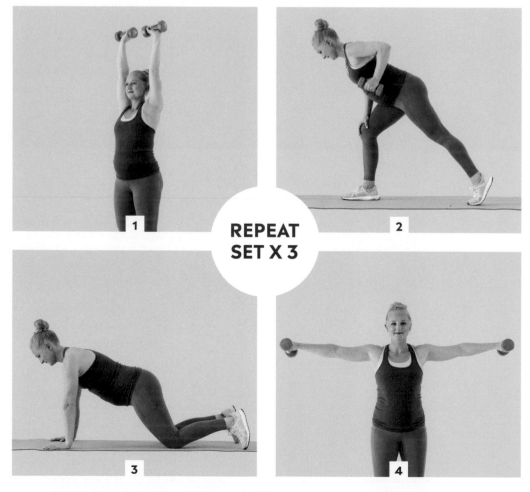

REPEAT SET X 3

CIRCUIT B

1. Bird dog x10 each side (p60)

2. Renegade row x10 alternating (p51)

3. Wide shoulder press x10 (p49)

4. Bicep curl x10 (p52)

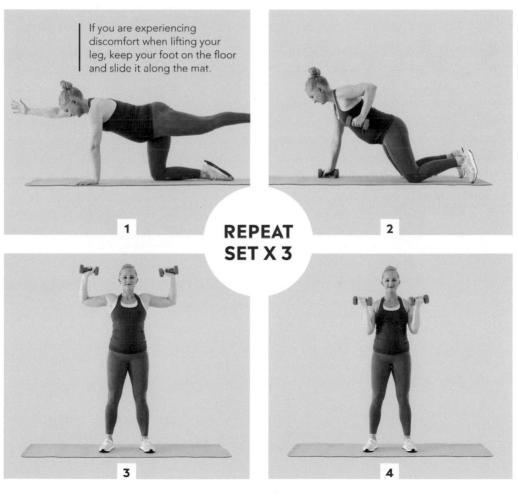

If you are experiencing discomfort when lifting your leg, keep your foot on the floor and slide it along the mat.

REPEAT SET X 3

UPPER BODY
WORKOUT 3

CIRCUIT A

1. Tricep extension x10 (p54)

2. Glute bridge chest press x10 (p56)

3. Wide shoulder press x10 (p49)

4. 4-point knee raise x5–10 (p61)

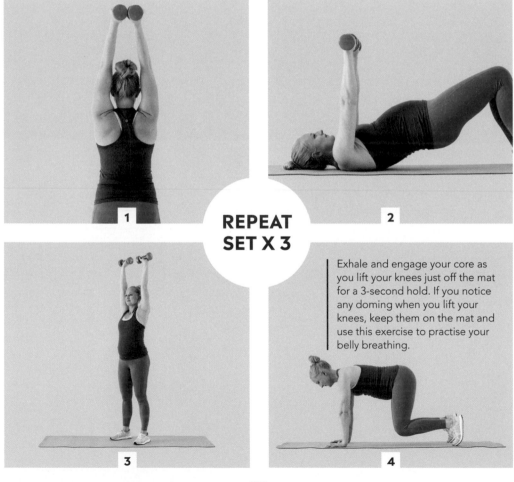

REPEAT SET X 3

Exhale and engage your core as you lift your knees just off the mat for a 3-second hold. If you notice any doming when you lift your knees, keep them on the mat and use this exercise to practise your belly breathing.

CIRCUIT B

1. Renegade row x10 alternating (p51)

2. Alternating shoulder press x20 (p48)

3. Glute bridge chest flye x10 (p57)

4. Arm raise x10 alternating (p47)

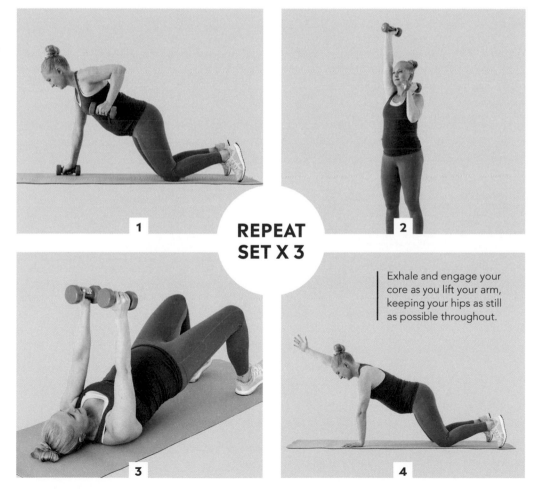

REPEAT SET X 3

Exhale and engage your core as you lift your arm, keeping your hips as still as possible throughout.

UPPER BODY
WORKOUT 4

CIRCUIT A

1. Narrow shoulder press x10 (p49)

2. Press-up x1 and 1 tap each shoulder x10 (p47)

3. Frontal & lateral raise x10 (p53)

4. Side plank crunch x10 each side (p59)

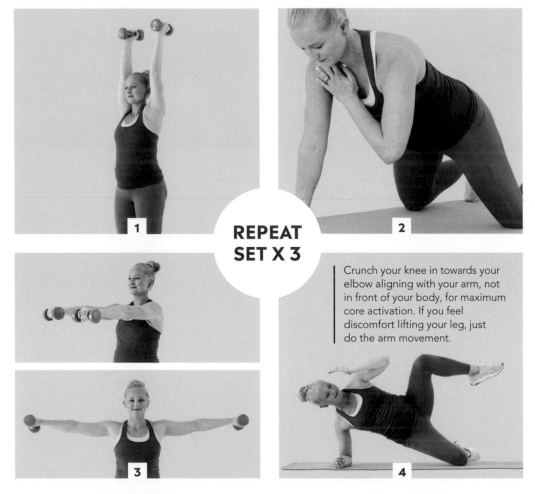

REPEAT SET X 3

Crunch your knee in towards your elbow aligning with your arm, not in front of your body, for maximum core activation. If you feel discomfort lifting your leg, just do the arm movement.

CIRCUIT B

1. Wide shoulder press x10 (p49)

2. Plank march x10 (p48)

3. Tricep dip x10 (p54)

4. Belly breathing x5 rounds (p61)

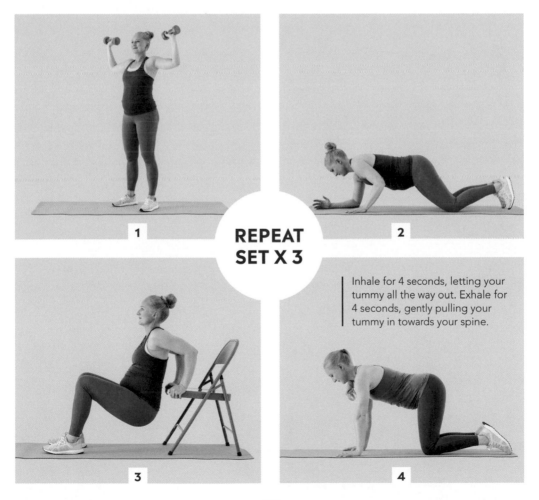

REPEAT SET X 3

Inhale for 4 seconds, letting your tummy all the way out. Exhale for 4 seconds, gently pulling your tummy in towards your spine.

LOWER BODY
WORKOUT 5

CIRCUIT A

1. Backward lunge x20 alternating (p38)

2. Good morning x10 (p41)

3. Glute bridge march x10–20 alternating (p44)

4. Bird dog x10 each side (p60)

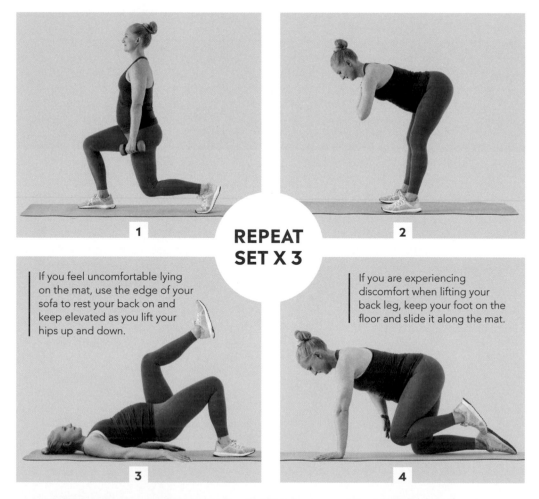

REPEAT SET X 3

If you feel uncomfortable lying on the mat, use the edge of your sofa to rest your back on and keep elevated as you lift your hips up and down.

If you are experiencing discomfort when lifting your back leg, keep your foot on the floor and slide it along the mat.

CIRCUIT B

1. Balance lunge x10 each side (p38)

2. Sumo squat x10 (p37)

3. Single glute bridge x10 each side (p43)

4. Side plank twist x10 each side (p58)

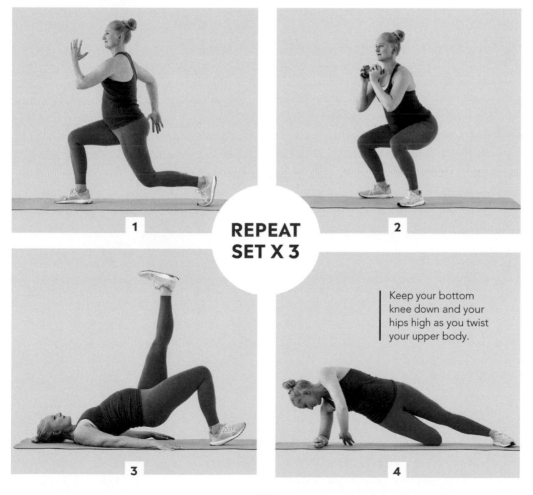

REPEAT SET X 3

Keep your bottom knee down and your hips high as you twist your upper body.

LOWER BODY
WORKOUT 6

CIRCUIT A

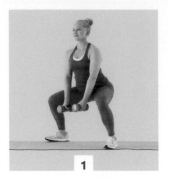
1

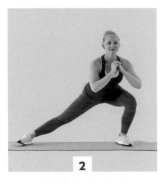

CIRCUIT A

1. Sumo deadlift x10 (p42)

2. Static side lunge x10 alternating (p40)

3. Lying leg crunch x10 each side (p45)

4. Side plank twist x10 each side (p58)

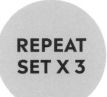
REPEAT SET X 3

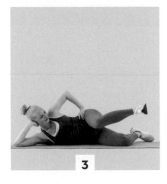
2

CIRCUIT B

1. Single RDL x10 each side (p42)

2. Sumo squat x10 (p37)

3. Glute bridge x10 (p43)

4. Shoulder tap x10 alternating (p60)

REPEAT SET X 3

3

Modified: Keep your bottom knee down and hips high as you twist your upper body.

4

CIRCUIT B

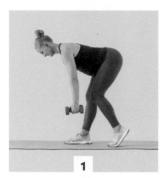

1

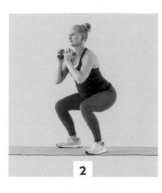

2

If you feel uncomfortable lying on the mat, use the edge of your sofa to rest your back on and keep elevated as you lift your hips up and down.

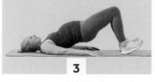

3

Take your time and keep your hips as still as possible.

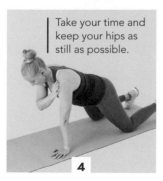

4

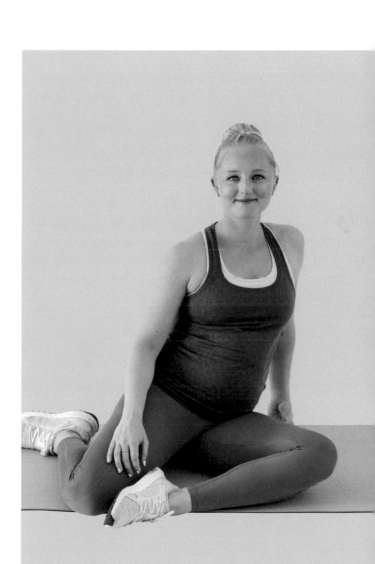

LOWER BODY
WORKOUT 7

CIRCUIT A

1. Sumo squat x15 (p37)

2. Side plank dip x10 each side (p59)

3. Reverse table top dip x10 (p46)

4. Lying leg raise x10 each side (p44)

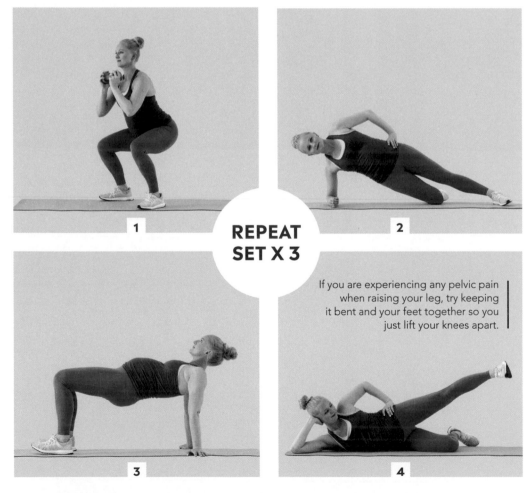

REPEAT SET X 3

If you are experiencing any pelvic pain when raising your leg, try keeping it bent and your feet together so you just lift your knees apart.

CIRCUIT B

1. Single glute bridge x10 each side (p43)

2. Romanian Deadlift (RDL) x10 (p41)

3. Balance lunge x10 each side (p38)

4. Shoulder tap x10–20 alternating (p60)

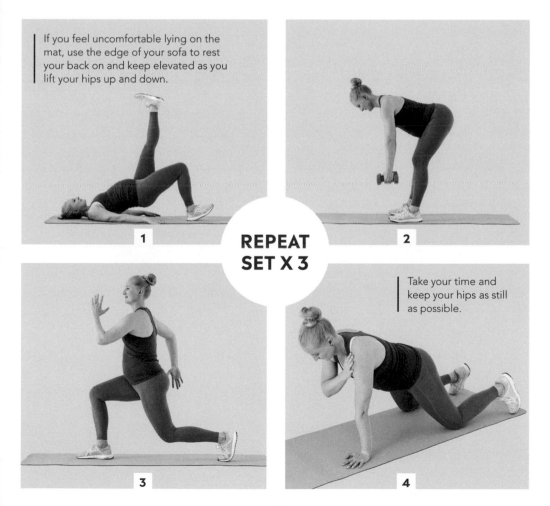

If you feel uncomfortable lying on the mat, use the edge of your sofa to rest your back on and keep elevated as you lift your hips up and down.

REPEAT
SET X 3

Take your time and keep your hips as still as possible.

LOWER BODY
WORKOUT 8

CIRCUIT A

1. Good morning x10 (p41)

2. Single glute bridge x10 each side (p43)

3. Single RDL x10 each side (p42)

4. Bird dog x10 each side (p60)

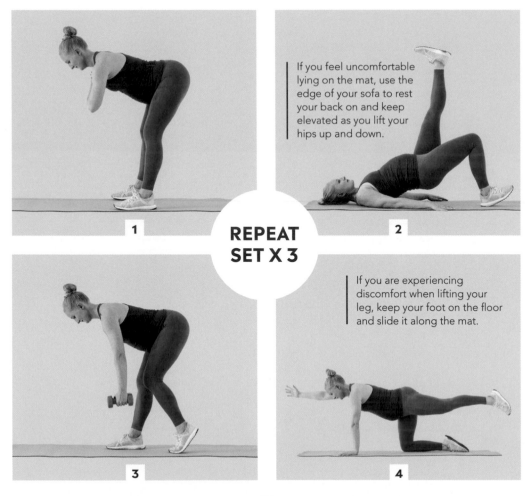

If you feel uncomfortable lying on the mat, use the edge of your sofa to rest your back on and keep elevated as you lift your hips up and down.

REPEAT SET X 3

If you are experiencing discomfort when lifting your leg, keep your foot on the floor and slide it along the mat.

CIRCUIT B

1. Pulsing squat 3 pulses x10 (p36)

2. Lying leg crunch x10 each side (p45)

3. Backward lunge x20 alternating (p38)

4. Side plank dip x10 each side (p59)

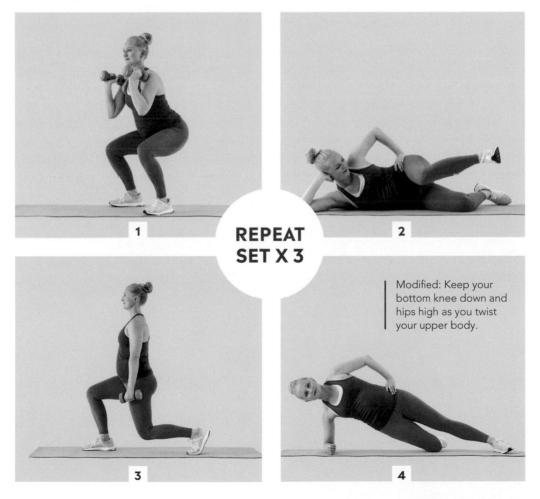

REPEAT SET X 3

1

2

Modified: Keep your bottom knee down and hips high as you twist your upper body.

3

4

FULL BODY
WORKOUT 9

CIRCUIT A

1. Squat & press x10 (p37)

2. Plank march x10 (p48)

3. Static lunge x10 each side (p39)

4. Reverse table top dip x10 (p46)

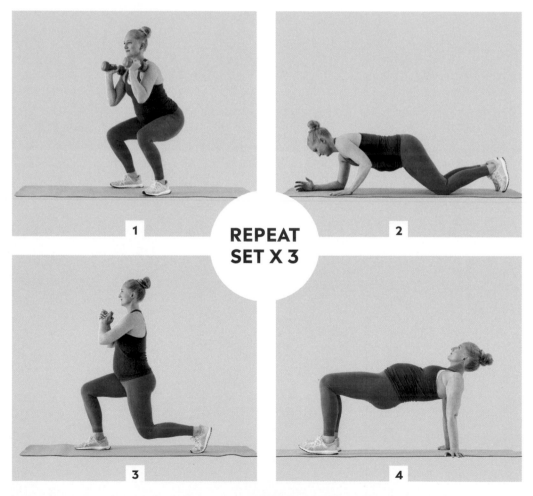

REPEAT
SET X 3

CIRCUIT B

1. Lunge & curl x20 alternating (p39)

2. Alternating shoulder press x10 (p48)

3. Side lunge x10 alternating (p40)

4. Arm raise x10 alternating (p47)

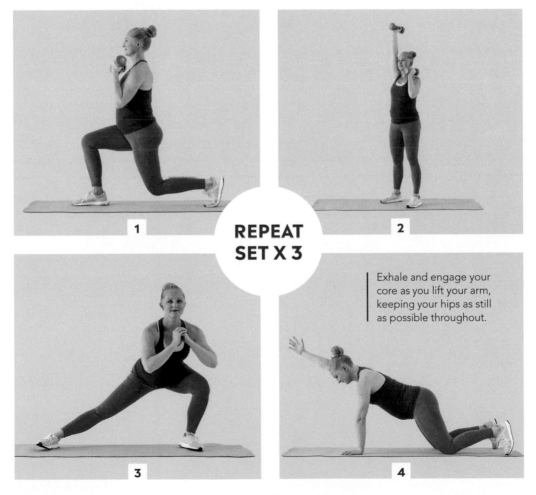

REPEAT SET X 3

Exhale and engage your core as you lift your arm, keeping your hips as still as possible throughout.

FULL BODY
WORKOUT 10

CIRCUIT A

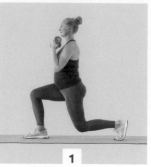

1. Lunge & curl x10 alternating (p39)

2. Press-up x1 and 1 tap each shoulder x10 (p47)

3. Squat & press x10 (p37)

4. Single bentover row x10 each side (p51)

REPEAT SET X 3

CIRCUIT B

1. Sumo squat x10 (p37)

2. Tricep dip x10 (p54)

3. Plank march x10 (p48)

4. Bird dog x10 each side (p60)

REPEAT SET X 3

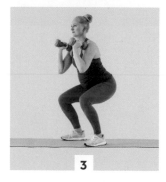

1

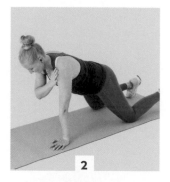

2

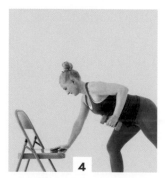

3

4

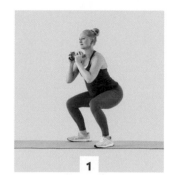

1

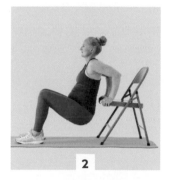

2

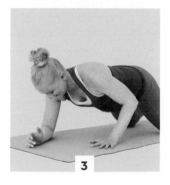

3

If you are experiencing discomfort when lifting your leg, keep your foot on the floor and slide it along the mat.

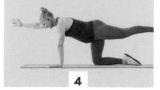

4

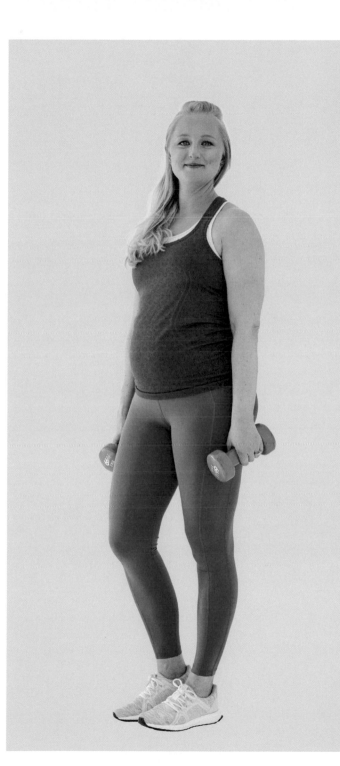

FULL BODY
WORKOUT 11

CIRCUIT A

1. Squat & press x10 (p37)

2. Bentover row x10 (p50)

3. Backward lunge x 20 alternating (p38)

4. Reverse table top dip x10 (p46)

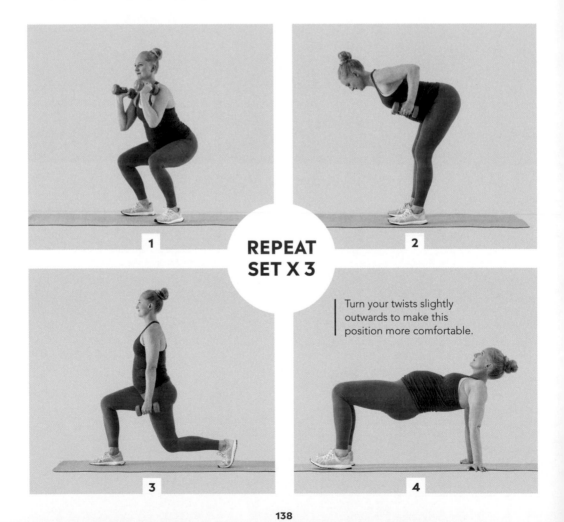

REPEAT SET X 3

Turn your twists slightly outwards to make this position more comfortable.

CIRCUIT B

1. Press-up x10 (p46)

2. Sumo squat x10 (p37)

3. Tricep dip x10 (p54)

4. Side plank twist x10 each side (p58)

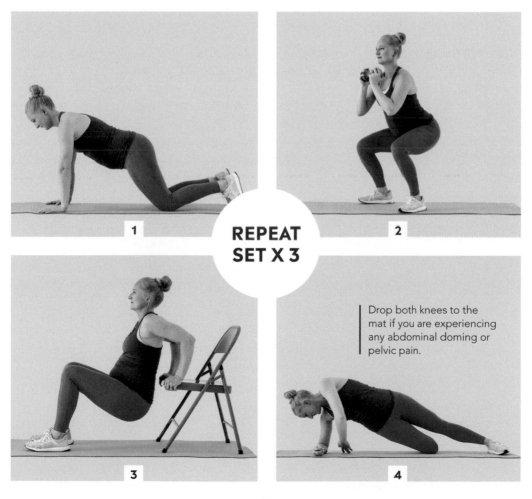

REPEAT SET X 3

Drop both knees to the mat if you are experiencing any abdominal doming or pelvic pain.

FULL BODY
WORKOUT 12

CIRCUIT A

1. Side lunge x10 alternating (p40)

2. Single bentover row x10 each side (p51)

3. Glute bridge chest press x10 (p56)

4. Arm raise x10 alternating (p47)

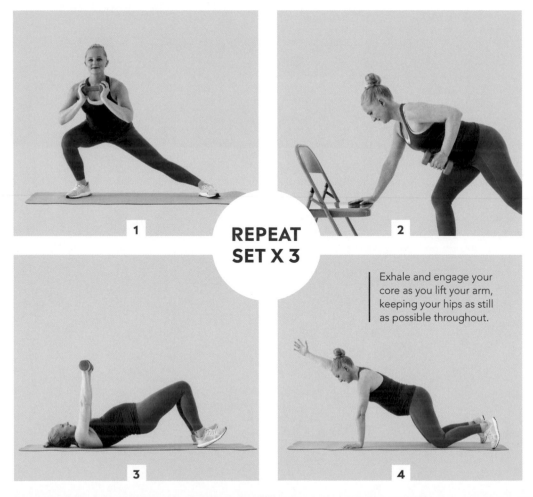

1

2

**REPEAT
SET X 3**

Exhale and engage your core as you lift your arm, keeping your hips as still as possible throughout.

3

4

CIRCUIT B

1. Squat & press x10 (p37)

2. Tricep extension x10 (p54)

3. Sumo deadlift x10 (p42)

4. Upright row x10 (p52)

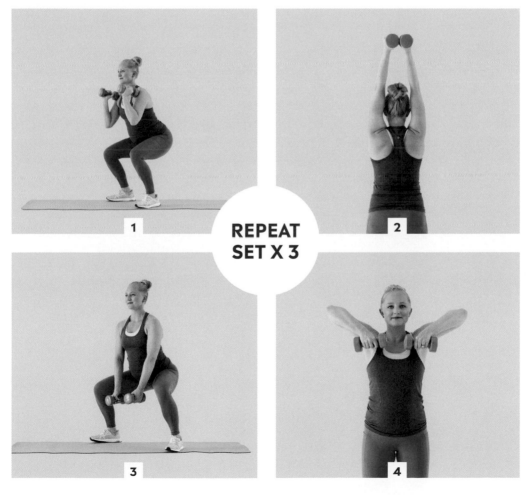

REPEAT
SET X 3

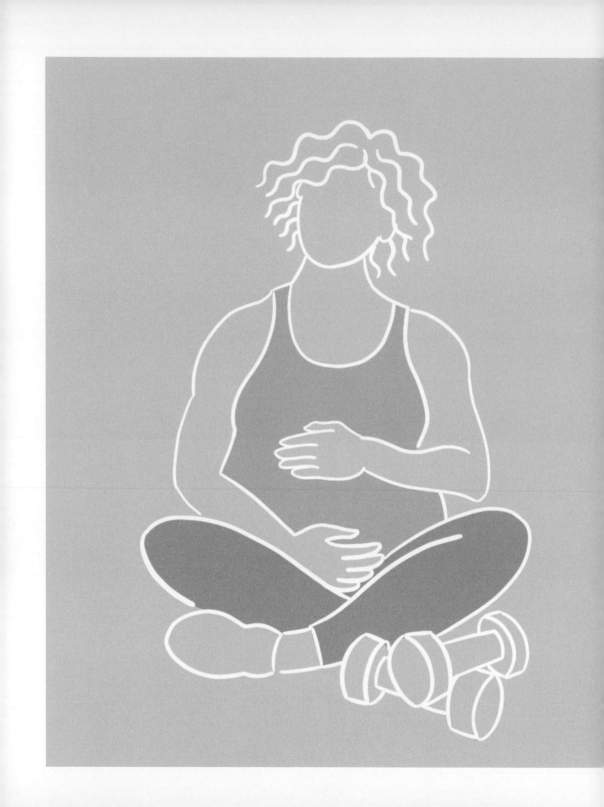

THIRD TRIMESTER

Weeks 28–40

You will tire more easily in the third trimester, as carrying the weight of your bump feels like a workout in itself. Self-care is the watch word as you get into the right frame of mind for labour and birth, and prepare for your baby's arrival.

WHAT TO EXPECT IN
THE THIRD TRIMESTER

Congratulations, you have made it to the third trimester. This starts from 28 weeks and takes you right up to the birth. You might find people saying to you, "Wow, your pregnancy has gone so fast" and, like me, you'll probably be thinking, "Erm, no it hasn't – I feel as though I've been pregnant for about a year already!" Don't worry if you don't feel like the pregnancy is flying by – I certainly didn't – but once I hit 28 weeks and entered into the third trimester, I did find that it started speeding up a little.

I couldn't believe I was in the third trimester, finally! Another big milestone.

MY BUMP WAS STILL RELATIVELY COMPACT UNTIL ABOUT WEEK 31 WHEN IT SEEMED TO DOUBLE IN SIZE OVERNIGHT – WELL NOT QUITE, BUT MY GOODNESS DID IT FEEL LIKE IT! ALL OF A SUDDEN I 'FELT PREGNANT'.

My bump was still relatively compact until about week 31, when it seemed to double in size overnight – well not quite, but my goodness did it feel like it! All of a sudden I 'felt pregnant' and got all sorts of niggly pains. Surely a personal trainer doesn't get pregnancy aches and pains you might be thinking… oh but she does, and she did!

ACHES AND PAINS

You can never predict how your body is going to react to pregnancy and even when doing all the things you are told to, you may still get some uncomfortable symptoms. I had some discomfort in my pelvis, which would come and go in the last few weeks, so I would always adapt my workouts to make sure they were comfortable for me and I followed the guidelines that are outlined in the first trimester (see page 69). My lower back would ache if I had been on my feet a lot, but other days I would feel fine. I had a delightful return of some pregnancy nausea. It was nowhere near

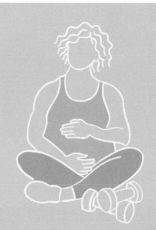

YOUR BABY AND BODY **IN THE THIRD TRIMESTER**

You and your baby may be two-thirds of the way there, but there is still plenty more growing to come, for you both. As your little one will be gaining a lot more weight from now to the birth, it will come as no surprise that the kicks and punches will start to become much bigger and more aggressive as time goes on. You will feel them up into your ribs and right down onto your bladder, which can be both exciting and inconvenient. The movement will go from sharp jabs to wriggles as the baby gets bigger, but remember he will never run out of room to move, so if you notice less movement at any time let your midwife know.

Your baby's bones will be hardening and he will take all his calcium from you. Make sure that your diet is rich in calcium, such as dairy foods and green leafy vegetables, so that you get a sufficient amount for yourself.

Your baby's skin is becoming less transparent and he is continuing to accumulate fat stores as he sheds his vernix, the white waxy substance that keeps him warm until there is enough fat to do the job.

At around 34 weeks, but sometimes later, your baby will make his way towards the pelvis, hopefully positioned head down and bottom up. As the head becomes engaged deeper into the pelvis, you may feel fewer kicks into your ribs and a bit more pressure in the pelvis and on your bladder. That is, of course, unless your baby is stubborn and decides not to get into this position, in which case your midwife will offer to try to turn him manually at around 37 weeks. Don't worry if your baby doesn't engage – you will still go into labour. My baby's head was engaged from 36 weeks and it meant nothing – I was still kept waiting beyond the due date!

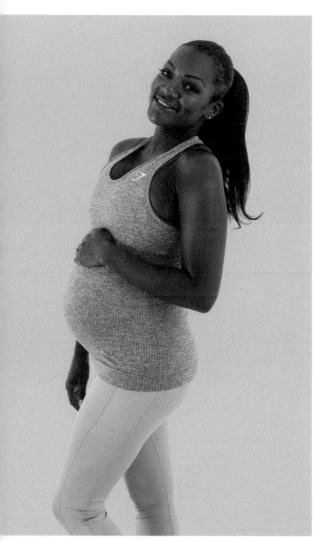

first trimester standards, but it took me by surprise until I realized that it could be solved by not letting myself get too hungry. Lesson quickly learned and snack cupboard stocked back up!

DIFFICULT DAYS

Pregnancy is incredible, and watching my body grow an actual human while I basically did nothing just blew my mind the whole way through. It didn't, however, mean that every day was wonderful. I'd had body image issues as a teenager and I was aware that I might struggle with my body changing during pregnancy. I managed to keep good control of my mental health overall, but there were a few days in the later weeks when it got the better of me.

As my bump was growing, I started feeling slower, heavier, and sometimes very uncomfortable. I got fed up on those days, not because I hated being pregnant – far from it – but because I wasn't used to the total and utter lack of control over my body. I was familiar with that full and heavy feeling after overeating on Christmas Day or after going out for a big meal, but now it was something I had to get used to daily.

I felt guilty about feeling down because I knew how long I'd waited to be pregnant, and I felt so incredibly lucky to be carrying our baby. George would kindly remind me that having an 'off day' didn't mean I wasn't grateful. It was always helpful to hear that.

> PREGNANCY IS ONE BIG EMOTIONAL ROLLERCOASTER. I SALUTE ALL PARTNERS FOR THE MULTIPLE TIMES YOU HAVE TO BITE YOUR TONGUE AND LET US JUST GET ON WITH IT.

'HORMOTIONAL' MOMENTS

The amount of hormones flying through your body in pregnancy often gets forgotten, but they can leave you with the most irrational thoughts and mood swings. I liked to call them 'hormotional moments', when you know you're being irrational but you simply can't help it!

An example of this was one afternoon when I was out walking and decided that I would go home and eat a wrap that I knew we had in the fridge. I was dreaming about this delicious lunch, only to walk through the door to see George finishing it off. Of course it wasn't his fault; I hadn't told him I wanted the wrap, and there was a fridge full of other food for me to eat, but I was livid. I didn't want anything else for lunch. I basically thanked him for making a pregnant woman starve – it was utterly ridiculous. I knew that deep down, but couldn't help those emotions coming out and the poor guy quickly rushed to the shops and bought me a wrap!

It was so silly, but I know I'm not the only one to have had moments like this, or to have burst into tears at an advert. Pregnancy is one big emotional rollercoaster. I salute all partners for the multiple times you have to bite your tongue and let us just get on with it.

EXERCISE IN THE
THIRD TRIMESTER

As with the other trimesters, there is a huge difference from the first week to the last week. For this reason, it is important to listen to your body throughout. Some days you will feel energetic and other days you'll have nothing to give and want to sleep all day. Both are normal.

At around week 31, I started to feel seriously heavy and noticed that I needed to slow down. Some mornings I would jump out of bed with a spring in my step and others I most definitely did not. Being the busy bee that I am, I found this more mentally tough than anything, but by organizing my week so that I knew when I could rest or have quieter days, I was able to schedule in my workouts accordingly.

BOSS BABY!

I learned the hard way that the baby is the boss, when I would sometimes try to fit too much into my day. When the baby needs more of your energy, he will just take it, leaving you with barely any, so on those days it is worth just letting that workout go and trying again the next day. This is a good habit to learn as it will come in very useful when the baby is earth side.

The bump is the main dictator of any exercise adaptations you need to make throughout pregnancy, and even more so now. Some exercises will just seem

> I LEARNED THE HARD WAY THAT THE BABY IS THE BOSS, WHEN I WOULD SOMETIMES TRY TO FIT TOO MUCH INTO MY DAY. WHEN THE BABY NEEDS MORE OF YOUR ENERGY, HE WILL JUST TAKE IT, LEAVING YOU WITH BARELY ANY.

physically impossible as your bump gets bigger and this will be different depending on your baby's position on that day, your other symptoms, and the tightness of your muscles, so pay attention to the signs your body is giving you. Touching, or even seeing, your toes may be out of the question soon, but there is still plenty that you can do, so don't give up just yet.

CARDIO EXERCISE

In the third trimester walking to the shops, let alone doing any shopping, can feel like cardio. I couldn't believe how doing the smallest of tasks tired me. Other days I would go for a walk and feel great, or spend half an hour on a spin bike and love it – it would just depend on the day and how my body was feeling at that time.

I always admired pregnant women who continued running with a bump. I just couldn't fathom it; the energy needed for that was beyond me, but well done to them! If you are still running, and feel comfortable doing so, then that's great. You just need to make sure you keep checking in with your body each and every time you go running. How do my hips feel? How does my pelvis feel? Can I catch my breath while I run? All these questions will allow you to keep assessing how happy your body is with running, and be very honest with yourself if and when it comes to putting it on hold for a while.

With any cardio in pregnancy, you need to be drinking plenty of water before, during, and after, as well as taking regular rests. This applies to everyone, at all stages in pregnancy, but even more so in your third trimester.

STRENGTH TRAINING

It is okay to continue to lift weights in your third trimester, as long as you feel fine doing so. Are you sick of me saying listen to your body yet? If you are still comfortable lifting the same weights that you have been using all along, then by all means carry on with them, but remember that 8–10 repetitions rule. If you are struggling to do 8–10 of any exercise, then there is always the option to lower the weights or even just use body weight. I know that it can feel like a mental loss for some of you – I also struggled with my competitive self – but now is the time to leave your ego at the door. Don't feel like you're failing by lowering your

DON'T FEEL LIKE YOU'RE FAILING BY LOWERING YOUR WEIGHTS. YOU ARE CARRYING AROUND A VERY WRIGGLY WEIGHT, ALL DAY EVERY DAY, WHICH IS GETTING HEAVIER – YOU ARE DEFINITELY NOT FAILING; YOU ARE ADAPTING.

weights. You are carrying around a very wriggly weight, all day every day, which is getting heavier – you are definitely not failing; you are adapting.

It is important to stretch alongside your strength training as a tight muscle is just as useless as a weak one. I know I bang on about keeping your muscles active to support your bump, but if you continually activate them, they are going to get very tight and end up causing other imbalances. Use the warm-up and cool down exercises on pages 26–33 as often as you can, whether you have exercised that day or not. You don't need to set aside a great deal of time – try doing a stretch when you're waiting for the kettle to boil, and another while the bath is running, then over the day you are getting to those important muscles.

YOUR CORE

You may be thinking, "What core?" as you near the end of your pregnancy. You can't see it and you probably can't feel it, but it is still in there working away to keep you upright. Your core is your entire middle, including your back and sides as well as your abdominals, and it has an important job supporting that bump

By 35 weeks almost all women will have an abdominal separation (see page 113), so you may be noticing a doming shape appear as you exercise or do daily activities. Use it as a guide to what is and isn't too much – if you see your core starting to create a 'pointy' shape, then that is your indicator to adapt or avoid that movement. Try using your breathing to control the tension (see page 75) during that exercise and if it still doesn't help, then move on.

PACKING YOUR
HOSPITAL BAG

When one of our antenatal class couples gave birth almost four weeks early, we swiftly got our butts into gear to pack our hospital bag! I went online and ordered it all – breastfeeding bras, nipple cream, maternity pads, giant knickers, scented sprays, mini fans, so many snacks...

I found packing the bag quite stressful if I'm honest. I wondered how long we would be in for? How hot would it be? How many nappies should I pack? What size babygro? I packed as if we might be in for a few days and I know I would unpack and repack multiple times before I actually went into labour, but at 34 weeks that bag was ready to go. We stood and stared at it, then at each other in excitement and anticipation, and left it by the front door. It felt like a big moment and that we really were ready!

One of the tips I found the most useful was to buy clear ziplock bags so that the contents of the hospital bag could be easily organized and hopefully easy for George to find. It is helpful to get your birth partner to pack the bag with you, so they have no excuse when you're demanding that mini-fan!

ITEMS **I ACTUALLY USED**

- Toothbrush and toothpaste
- Deodorant
- Face wipes
- Dry shampoo
- Vaseline
- Breastfeeding bras
- Nipple pads
- Disposable pants
- Flip-flops
- George's button-up shirt
- Pillow
- Muslins
- Babygros
- Cotton hat
- Warm hooded top for the baby
- Cellular blanket
- Nappies
- Wipes

PLANNING FOR THE BIRTH
MENTALLY

Planning for the birth is like planning for a holiday, except you're not sure exactly when you're leaving, what the weather is going to be like, how long you're staying for, and what will happen when you're there. It can feel very daunting. Some women want to know absolutely everything about labour and birth, and some as little as is necessary. I fell more into the first camp.

Eager to learn, I signed myself and George up for an antenatal class where we met with eight other couples; they were all due around the same time as us and lived fairly close by. We were really lucky and got on well with everyone in our group – it didn't feel forced at all. It was nice that we had one huge thing in common and we were all there to find out the same things. I went in naively thinking that I would know a lot of it because I had worked with pregnant women for so many years, but was quickly proven wrong as we discussed every little eventuality in detail, and so much of it I hadn't known.

I found it hard to sleep on the nights after our classes as my brain was full to the brim with information, but the more I learnt, the more empowered and ready I felt. Doing the classes with George was helpful as we were learning together. Well, mostly! He was very surprised to learn how many nappies a newborn would get through in a day, claiming he thought maybe two or three would be the maximum! We learnt about the different stages and options in labour and how to prepare to come home with a newborn. There were lots of dropped jaws from partners during the labour sections and nods from the mums-to-be as if to say, "See, this is what I am going to have to go through!" One of the main things that kept coming up was that we had a choice in everything; nothing

> THERE WERE LOTS OF DROPPED JAWS FROM PARTNERS DURING THE LABOUR SECTIONS AND NODS FROM THE MUMS-TO-BE AS IF TO SAY, "SEE, THIS IS WHAT I AM GOING TO HAVE TO GO THROUGH!"

would be done without our permission. This is important to remember throughout your pregnancy – always ask questions; write them down before appointments if you need to. By being well-informed, you can make the right decisions for you and your baby on the day. Making a birth plan can be useful, but think of it as preferences rather than a rigid plan – things can change in an instant, so it is important to be open to other options.

We bought some pregnancy books, and were given some, all of which sat on our bedside tables and looked very promising for weeks on end. Sound familiar? My advice – read the books that you want to read, but don't feel guilty for the ones you don't get around to.

HYPNOBIRTHING

A number of people recommended hypnobirthing – they swore that it was the sole reason they had a great birth, so I was very intrigued by it. I loved the idea of being able to "breathe my baby out with no pain" – I mean who wouldn't?

This was until I realized that this wasn't exactly the promise of hypnobirthing. The idea is to stay in control of your emotions by knowing exactly what is going on in your body, and remain calm in situations that could potentially become stressful, in all eventualities of birth. It is a mixture of breathing techniques and visualization.

I listened to audio tracks of relaxation techniques and affirmations that I planned to take with me when birthing my baby, and I found them really calming. I tried to get George to listen to them too, but he would be fast asleep within minutes – not ideal, but I figured that if they relaxed us enough to have a good night's sleep, then that couldn't be a bad thing. I loved the idea that the body knows what it's doing in birth; I found it really empowering and it gave me confidence in myself.

Having said that, remember that this is your pregnancy and just because the lady down the road swears by hypnobirthing, it might not be for you. Don't feel pressure to do anything that doesn't feel right for you.

PLANNING FOR THE BIRTH
PHYSICALLY

As my due date approached, I found myself worrying about whether I'd be able to cope with labour and birth. I like to be proactive so I tried to prepare my body physically. I didn't know whether what I tried would work, but I felt like I was doing something positive and that felt good. I tried perineal massage, pelvic floor relaxation, and stretching to keep my body feeling as loose as it could.

PERINEAL MASSAGE

Some women will do perineal massage to prevent tearing and some just can't face it. Here are the facts so you can decide for yourself.

Perineal massage is the focused stretching of the perineum (the area between the vaginal opening and the back passage) in the weeks running up to the birth. It is advised that all women are educated about its use from 35 weeks. By gradually stretching the skin, connective tissue, and muscles, you can reduce the risk of episiotomy and tears; the risk of third- or fourth-degree tears; experience less perineal pain; have better wound healing; reduce the length of the pushing stage of labour; and reduce the risk of bowel incontinence. Here's how to do it:

1. Wash your hands, then apply lubricant to the vulva and vaginal opening. Insert approximately 2.5cm (1in) of your thumb into your vagina.
2. Visualize a clock – 12 at the pubic bone and 6 at the anus (see opposite) to help you to work systematically.
3. Start with gentle sweeping motions from 3–9 o'clock, to get used to the stretching sensations, then apply pressure down towards the anus (ie. 6 o'clock) and hold for around 30 seconds. You can repeat this for all areas between 3–9 o'clock. Breathe slowly and calmly whilst doing this. You should feel pressure and stretching, but not pain.

Start gently and increase the pressure as the weeks go on. You may want to use both thumbs to stretch both sides at the same time as you progress and feel more confident. Aim for 5–10 minutes once or twice per week.

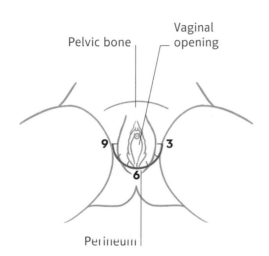

Pelvic bone

Vaginal opening

9 3

6

Perineum

PERINEAL MASSAGE

Caution: Do not perform perineal massage if you have any vaginal bleeding, active infections, or ruptured membranes. If you have any concerns, check with your midwife or GP first.

RELAXED PELVIC FLOOR

Now more than ever it is important to focus on deep breathing and letting your pelvic floor let go and relax, making sure

not to hold the muscles tightly. The pelvic floor needs to be strong but flexible for birth; the muscles need to relax to enable them to go through the full range of motion. Research shows that there isn't an increased risk of tearing from doing pelvic floor muscle exercises in pregnancy.

So when you are doing your pelvic floor exercises, breathe deeply between each one, and regularly breathe deeply into the base of your ribs and tummy. So many of us hold our pelvic floor and tummy tight. Having grown up doing gymnastics and a high level of impact training, my pelvic floor was in a state of constant tightness, so I had to work really hard to relax it.

DIASTASIS

Remember to keep an eye out for the signs of diastasis (see pages 113–114) during exercise and your day-to-day life (and know that you are not alone, and haven't done anything wrong for this to occur). Those muscles have stretched to allow your baby to grow up to this point, which is amazing and unavoidable!

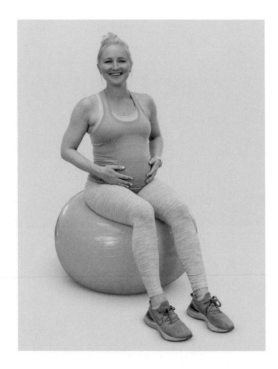

AS WE KNOW BY NOW, THE BABY IS THE BOSS AND HE WILL DO WHAT HE LIKES, BUT THERE ARE A FEW THINGS YOU CAN TRY TO ENCOURAGE HIM INTO AN OPTIMAL POSITION.

way. Firstly, he can move right up until the day he arrives, but also midwives and doctors are brilliant at helping to move the baby into an optimal position before or even during labour. As we know by now, the baby is the boss and he will do what he likes, but there are a few things you can try to encourage him into the optimal position.

YOUR BABY'S POSITION

The ideal birthing position for your baby is anterior, which means head down, with his back against your tummy. An optimal foetal position can contribute to the labour being quicker and less painful, which is obviously the goal, but don't panic if your baby is facing a different

Use a birthing ball

This is essentially a large exercise ball that you may find in the gym; they are relatively inexpensive and can be bought online for you to pump up at home. The ball can replace your chair at the dinner table, your office chair, and even your sofa towards the end of pregnancy. It will become your best friend as it is extremely helpful for encouraging the baby to move down into the pelvic area, hopefully head first.

A birthing ball is also great for helping you sit with good posture, rather than slumping into the sofa, which will become less and less comfortable and harder and harder to get up from. Sitting on the ball and gently bouncing, or making figures of eight with your hips, will help to keep your pelvis open and give your baby the best possible chance of nestling in there.

It is really useful during labour too, so even though they are big and a pain to store anywhere when blown up, they're worth having around in the final stage of pregnancy.

Don't cross your legs

At my 32-week appointment, my midwife instructed me to stop sitting or standing with my legs crossed. She said that this would close off my pelvis, making it harder for my baby to get into position. I thought it would be easy as I was sure

I didn't cross my legs too often, but it's crazy how many times I would find myself sitting or standing with crossed legs. Get your partner to keep an eye out for this too and encourage you to sit in an unladylike way with your legs apart.

Get onto your hands and knees

A handy way to use gravity to help your baby move into a good position for birth is to position yourself on all-fours for 10 minutes twice a day. You can use this time to stretch your back out, or focus on some breathing techniques (see page 75 for using a breathing exercise as part of your workout).

Keep your hips above your knees

Collapsing into very soft sofas and armchairs can seem very appealing when you're exhausted, but the reality is that when your hips sink lower than your knees, it closes off your pelvis and doesn't leave a huge amount of room for your baby to make his way in. Pile up some cushions to keep you sitting higher than your knees, or use your birthing ball instead.

GOING
OVERDUE

Going overdue is something I wasn't mentally prepared for, and it turned out to be one of the most challenging parts of pregnancy for me.

From the second you see that positive pregnancy test, you will have done all the maths and found out your estimated due date. No matter how many times the midwife tells you it's an estimation, it is still the date that you work towards in your head. That is the day my baby will come, and no plans will exist after then! In fact, only about 4 per cent of babies arrive on their due date. The full-term window is from 37 to 42 weeks, which is a huge and very vague amount of time. This is why some women decide not to tell anyone their due date, simply their due month, because it takes the pressure off that specific date.

FINDING WAYS TO RELAX

Many women find this time tough, understandably; it's like waiting for a ticking time bomb to go off. You don't want to go too far from home, but you want to keep busy to distract yourself from over-analysing every single symptom that you feel. Was that a contraction? Has my bump dropped? It can feel very stressful and, of course, everyone tells you to relax, which is unhelpful when you're feeling the opposite! They are right, though – for all the old wives' tales about ways to bring on labour, any midwife will tell you that being relaxed is the most effective way to do it. It can help to feel like you are

EVERYONE TELLS YOU TO RELAX, WHICH IS UNHELPFUL WHEN YOU'RE FEELING THE OPPOSITE!

doing something proactive, but who knows if any of it helps. The baby will come when it is ready to and, unfortunately, that is not up to us to decide. You can eat all the spicy curries you like, drink raspberry leaf tea, eat 10 dates a day, or even attempt heavily pregnant sex to get the baby moving, but staying relaxed works best.

Relaxing doesn't have to involve lying in a bath with scented candles all around you; if you're not a bath person, then this won't feel relaxing. Just spend time doing things you enjoy, and that might be going for a walk, listening to some nice music, having a cup of tea with a friend, or even baking a cake.

BEING ACTIVE

Staying active can help to bring on labour, as long as you don't overdo it. You don't want to go into labour with aching muscles. You want to feel energized and limber, so that you can move in a way that will help you to feel comfortable through your contractions. I would advise lowering the weights you use in those last few weeks, if you use any at all; your bump is plenty of weight to be carrying around.

Go for walks at a leisurely pace; if your baby is sitting low, then this is probably all that you can manage comfortably. Sit on that birthing ball (see page 156) at home to allow your pelvis to stay as open as possible and encourage your baby to

TEXT **STRESS**

You might feel like throwing your phone out of the window with the amount of texts you're getting from family and friends. They can't help getting excited, but it can really get on your nerves. Politely let them know that as soon as there is news you will tell them, and remind them that you want this baby to come just as much as they do, and funnily enough probably even more!

move down into the 'departure lounge' if he isn't already. It can also provide a comfortable position to sit in, because sitting slumped on a sofa may no longer be ideal with the baby getting up close and personal to your ribs and bladder at the same time!

Try to ensure you're not in the same position for too long; move about every so often to keep the blood flowing and prevent you from feeling stiff and achy.

THIRD TRIMESTER
WORKOUT PLAN

The difference in size between your bump at the beginning of this trimester and the end will differ hugely. This change will alter your workouts, whether it is the weights you choose, the number of breaks you take, or the pace at which you do them. There are 12 workouts in this section and the instructions for each can be found in the Pose Directory on pages 36–61. You'll see some more adaptations that will further allow for your growing bump, taking the pressure off your core whilst keeping it engaged still.

As your bump becomes heavier, you may feel that you want to lower your weights or just stick mainly to body weight. Don't forget, you already have a permanent weight attached to your front so you're doing just fine! You know your body better than anyone else – do what feels right for you and you might even decide that you want to stop these workouts a few weeks before your due date. Make sure to add lots of stretching into your week as well – see the Warm Up & Cool Down section on pages 26–33.

UPPER BODY
WORKOUT 1

CIRCUIT A

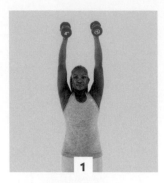

1. Narrow shoulder press x10 (p49)

2. Bentover row x10 (p50)

3. Press-up x10 (p46)

4. Shoulder tap x10 alternating (p60)

REPEAT SET X 3

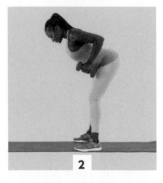

CIRCUIT B

1. Lateral raise x10 (p53)

2. Tricep extension x10 (p54)

3. Plank march x10 (p48)

4. Side plank twist x10 each side (p58)

REPEAT SET X 3

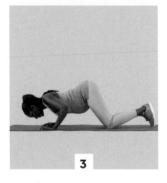

Keep your knees wide and your hips as still as possible as you lift your arms.

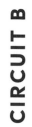

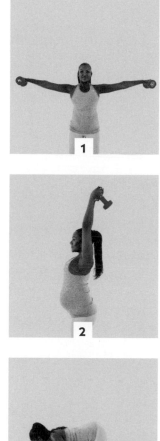

1

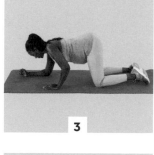

2

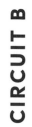

3

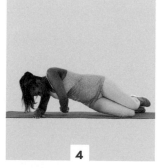

4

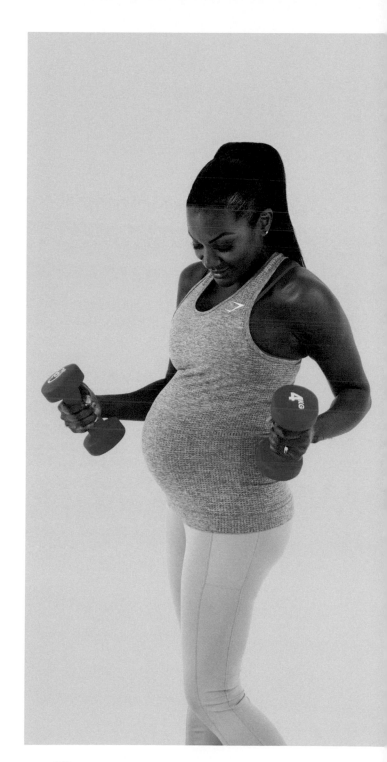

UPPER BODY
WORKOUT 2

CIRCUIT A

1. Alternating shoulder press x10 (p48)

2. Frontal raise x10 (p53)

3. Curl & press x10 (p50)

4. Shoulder tap x10 alternating (p60)

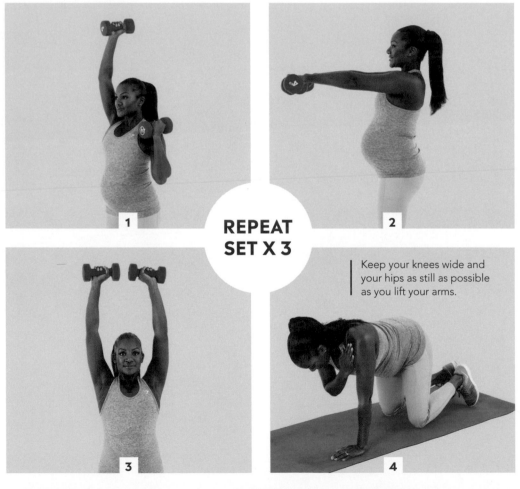

REPEAT SET X 3

Keep your knees wide and your hips as still as possible as you lift your arms.

CIRCUIT B

1. Bentover row x10 (p50)

2. Bicep curl x10 (p52)

3. Glute bridge chest press x10 (p56)

4. Bird dog x10 each side (p60)

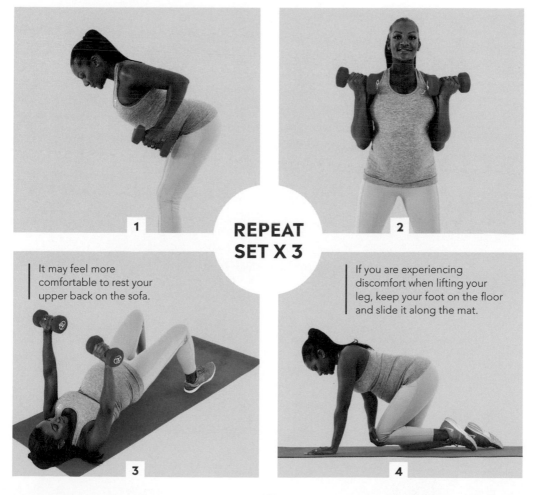

REPEAT SET X 3

1

2

It may feel more comfortable to rest your upper back on the sofa.

If you are experiencing discomfort when lifting your leg, keep your foot on the floor and slide it along the mat.

3

4

UPPER BODY
WORKOUT 3

CIRCUIT A

1. Alternating shoulder press x10 (p48)

2. Press-up x10 (p46)

3. Lateral raise x10 (p53)

4. Bird dog x10 each side (p60)

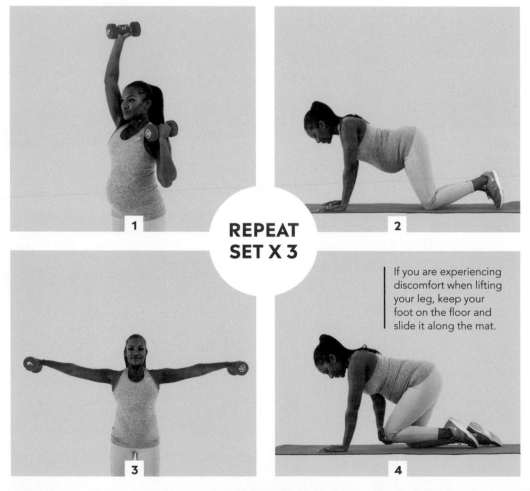

REPEAT
SET X 3

If you are experiencing discomfort when lifting your leg, keep your foot on the floor and slide it along the mat.

CIRCUIT B

1. Bicep curl x10 (p52)

2. Single bentover row x10 each side (p51)

3. Tricep extension x10 (p54)

4. Arm raise x10 (p47)

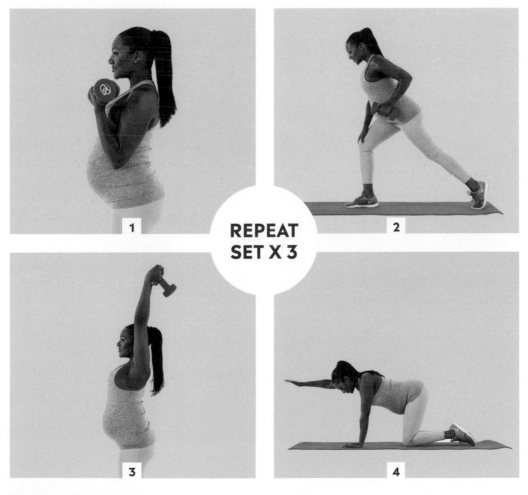

REPEAT SET X 3

UPPER BODY
WORKOUT 4

CIRCUIT A

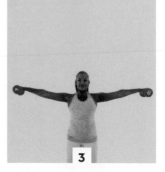

CIRCUIT A

1. Single bentover row
x10 each side (p51)

2. Narrow shoulder press
x10 (p49)

3. Lateral raise x10 (p53)

4. Tricep extension x10 (p54)

REPEAT SET X 3

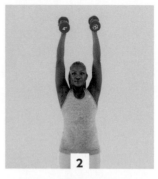

CIRCUIT B

1. Press-up x10 (p46)

2. Frontal raise x10 (p53)

3. Wide shoulder press (p49)

4. Shoulder tap x10 alternating
(p60)

REPEAT SET X 3

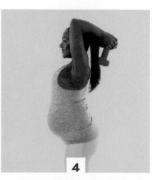

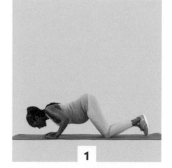

1

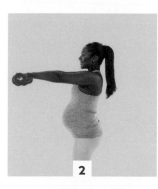

2

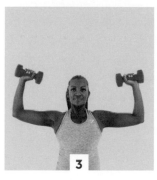

3

Keep your knees wide and your hips as still as possible as you lift your arms.

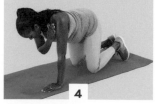

4

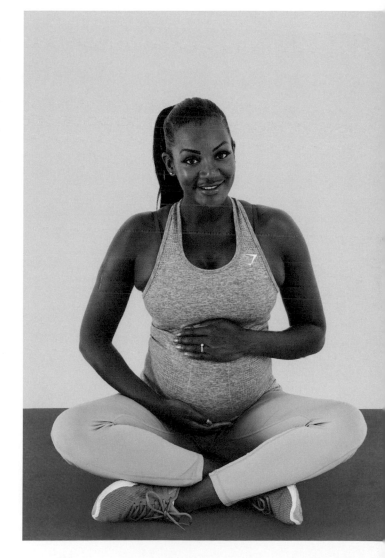

LOWER BODY
WORKOUT 5

CIRCUIT A

1. Squat & press x10 (p37)

2. Side lunge x10 alternating (p40)

3. Lying leg crunch x10 each side (p45)

4. Side plank twist x10 each side (p58)

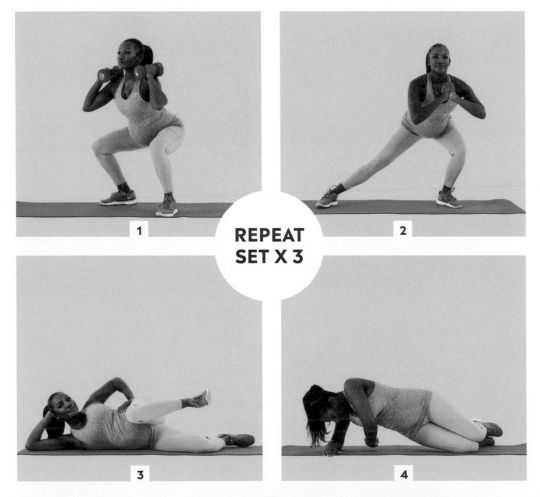

REPEAT SET X 3

1

2

3

4

CIRCUIT B

1. Balance lunge x10 each side (p38)

2. Sumo squat x10 (p37)

3. Glute bridge x10 (p43)

4. Lying leg raise x10 each side (p44)

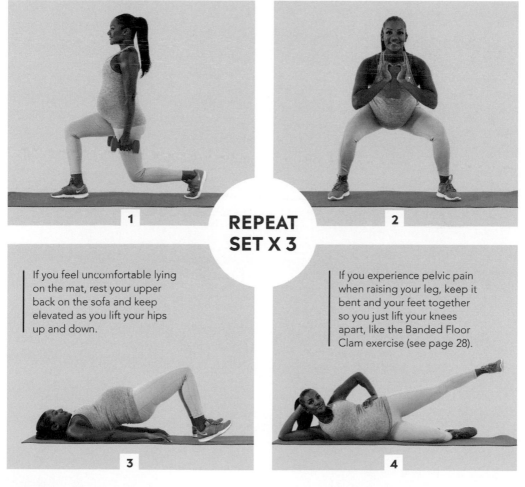

REPEAT SET X 3

If you feel uncomfortable lying on the mat, rest your upper back on the sofa and keep elevated as you lift your hips up and down.

If you experience pelvic pain when raising your leg, keep it bent and your feet together so you just lift your knees apart, like the Banded Floor Clam exercise (see page 28).

LOWER BODY
WORKOUT 6

CIRCUIT A

1. Sumo deadlift x10 (p42)

2. Backward lunge x10 alternating (p38)

3. Glute bridge x10 (p43)

4. Side plank twist x10 each side (p58)

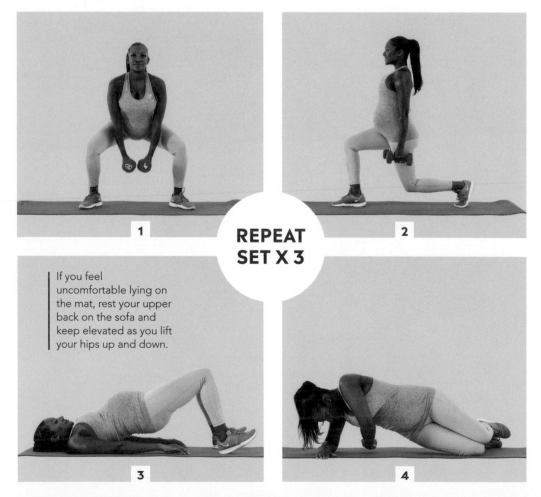

REPEAT
SET X 3

If you feel uncomfortable lying on the mat, rest your upper back on the sofa and keep elevated as you lift your hips up and down.

CIRCUIT B

1. Squat & press x10 (p37)

2. Bird dog x10 each side (p60)

3. Romanian Deadlift (RDL) x10 (p41)

4. Belly breathing x5 rounds (p61)

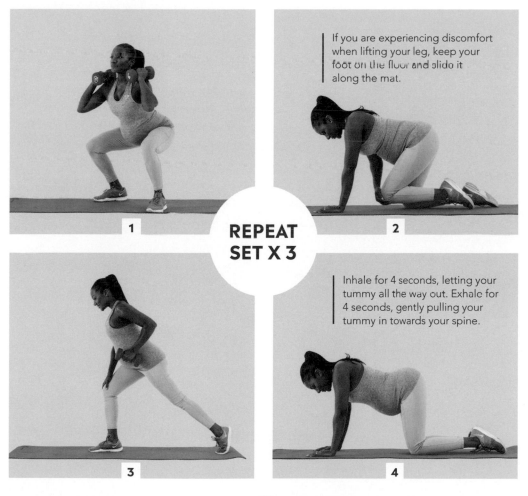

If you are experiencing discomfort when lifting your leg, keep your foot on the floor and slide it along the mat.

REPEAT SET X 3

Inhale for 4 seconds, letting your tummy all the way out. Exhale for 4 seconds, gently pulling your tummy in towards your spine.

LOWER BODY
WORKOUT 7

CIRCUIT A

1. Romanian Deadlift (RDL) x10 (p41)

2. Glute bridge march x10 (p44)

3. Squat & press x10 (p37)

4. Lying leg raise x10 each side (p44)

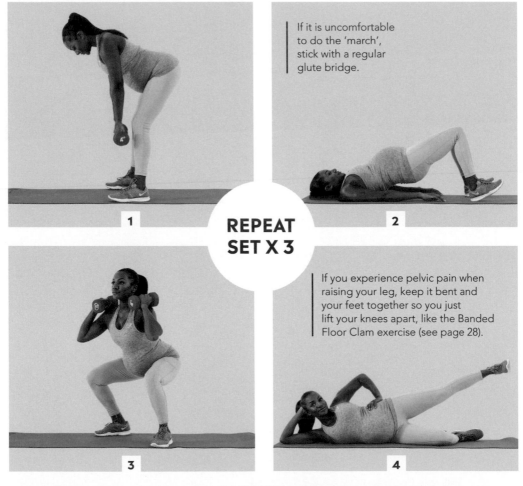

If it is uncomfortable to do the 'march', stick with a regular glute bridge.

REPEAT SET X 3

If you experience pelvic pain when raising your leg, keep it bent and your feet together so you just lift your knees apart, like the Banded Floor Clam exercise (see page 28).

1

2

3

4

CIRCUIT B

1. Single RDL x10 each side (p42)

2. Sumo squat x10 (p37)

3. Side plank dip x10 each side (p59)

4. Shoulder tap x10 alternating (p60)

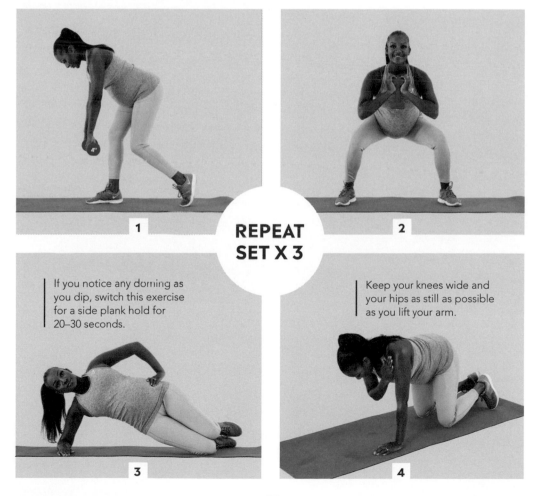

REPEAT SET X 3

If you notice any doming as you dip, switch this exercise for a side plank hold for 20–30 seconds.

Keep your knees wide and your hips as still as possible as you lift your arm.

LOWER BODY
WORKOUT 8

CIRCUIT A

1. Squat & press x10 (p37)

2. Static lunge x10 each side (p39)

3. Glute bridge x10 (p43)

4. Bird dog x10 each side (p60)

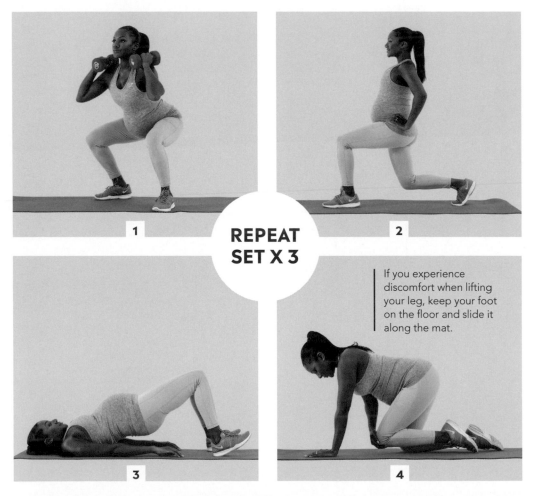

REPEAT SET X 3

If you experience discomfort when lifting your leg, keep your foot on the floor and slide it along the mat.

CIRCUIT B

1. Sumo squat x10 (p37)

2. Side plank twist x10 each side (p58)

3. Side lunge x10 alternating (p40)

4. Belly breathing x5 rounds (p61)

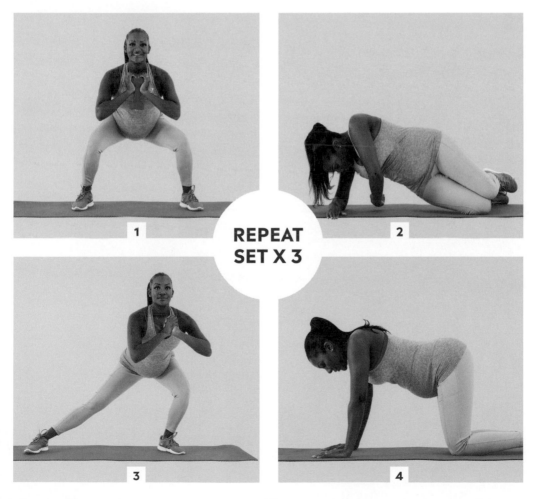

REPEAT SET X 3

FULL BODY
WORKOUT 9

CIRCUIT A

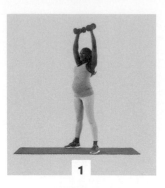

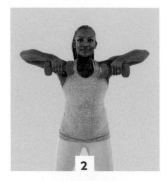

CIRCUIT A

1. Squat & press x10 (p37)

2. Upright row x10 (p52)

3. Static lunge x10 each side (p39)

4. Arm raise x10 alternating (p47)

REPEAT SET X 3

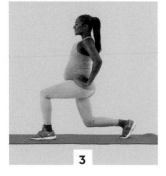

CIRCUIT B

1. Press-up x10 (p46)

2. Pulsing squat 3 pulses x10 (p36)

3. Bentover row x10 (p50)

4. Side plank x20–30 seconds each side (p58)

REPEAT SET X 3

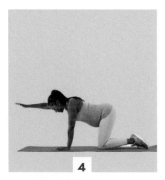

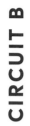

CIRCUIT B

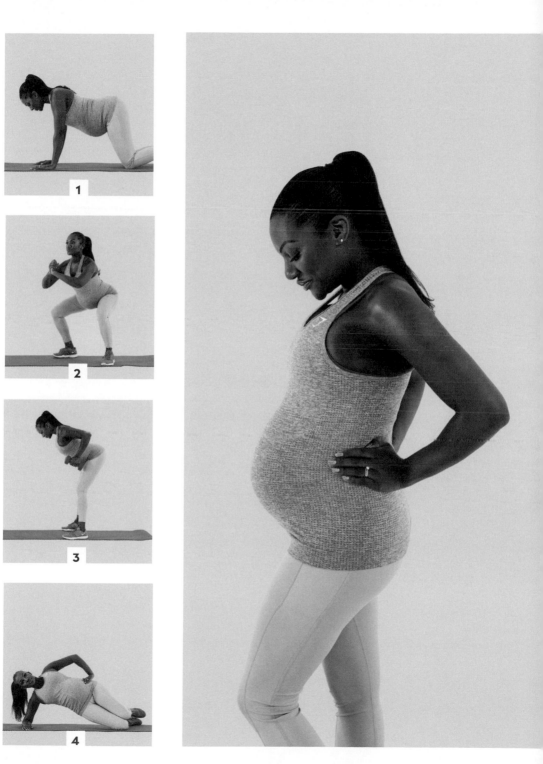

1

2

3

4

179

FULL BODY
WORKOUT 10

CIRCUIT A

1. Lunge & curl x10 alternating (p39)

2. Frontal & lateral raise x10 (p53)

3. Sumo deadlift x10 (p42)

4. Narrow shoulder press x10 (p49)

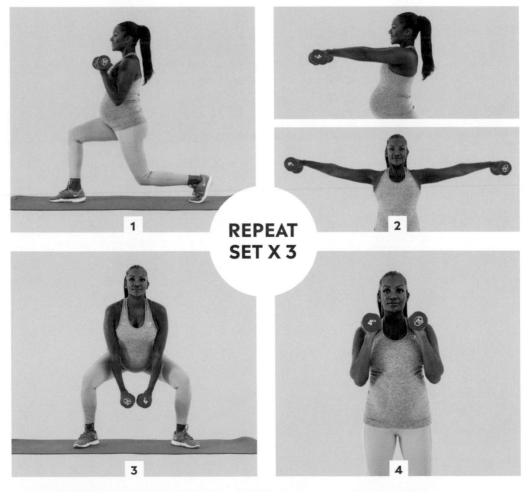

REPEAT SET X 3

1

2

3

4

CIRCUIT B

1. Press-up x1 and 1 tap each shoulder x10 (p47)

2. Pulsing squat 3 pulses x10 (p36)

3. Wide shoulder press x10 (p49)

4. Arm raise x10 alternating (p47)

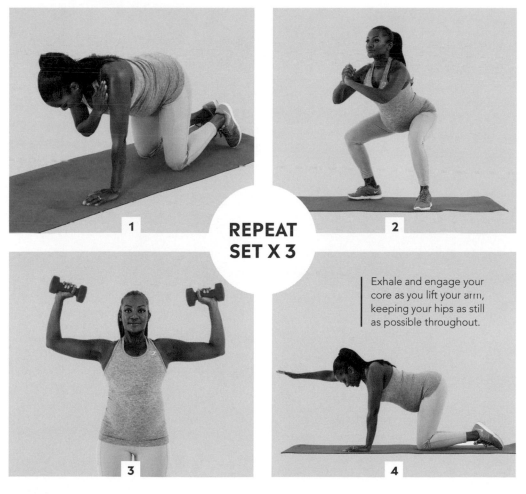

REPEAT SET X 3

Exhale and engage your core as you lift your arm, keeping your hips as still as possible throughout.

FULL BODY
WORKOUT 11

CIRCUIT A

1. Squat & press x10 (p37)

2. Upright row x10 (p52)

3. Curl & press x10 (p50)

4. Side lunge x10 alternating (p40)

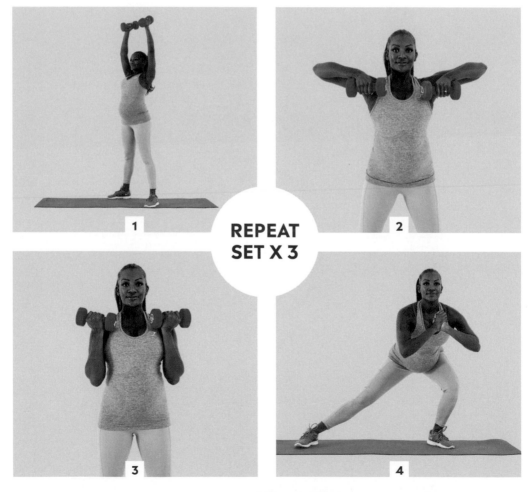

REPEAT
SET X 3

CIRCUIT B

1. Balance lunge x10 alternating (p38)

2. Arm raise x10 alternating (p47)

3. Sumo deadlift x10 (p42)

4. Glute bridge chest press x10 (p56)

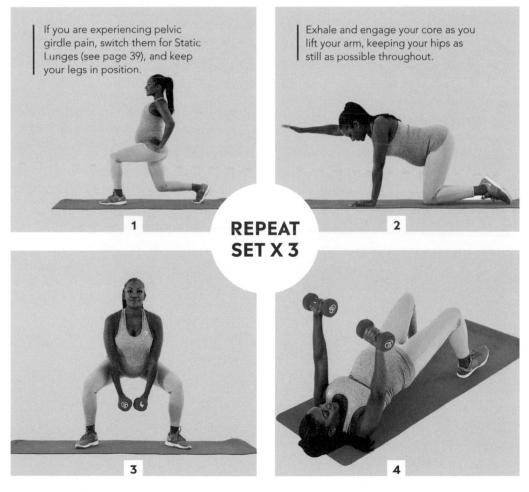

If you are experiencing pelvic girdle pain, switch them for Static Lunges (see page 39), and keep your legs in position.

Exhale and engage your core as you lift your arm, keeping your hips as still as possible throughout.

REPEAT SET X 3

FULL BODY
WORKOUT 12

CIRCUIT A

1. Lunge & curl x10 alternating (p39)

2. Alternating shoulder press x10–20 (p48)

3. Pulsing squat 3 pulses x10 (p36)

4. Side plank x20–30 seconds each side (p58)

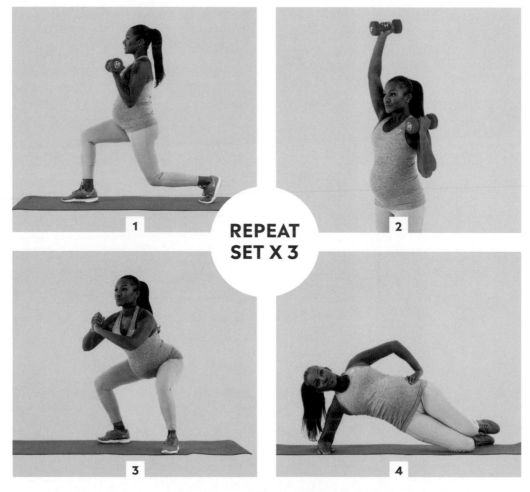

REPEAT SET X 3

CIRCUIT B

1. Plank march x10 (p48)

2. Squat & press x10 (p37)

3. Upright row x10 (p52)

4. Side lunge x10 alternating (p40)

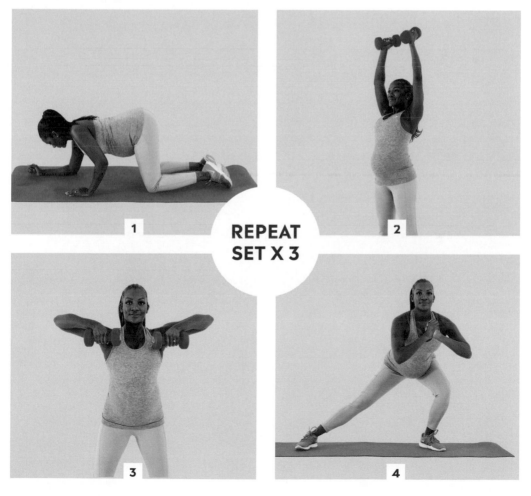

REPEAT SET X 3

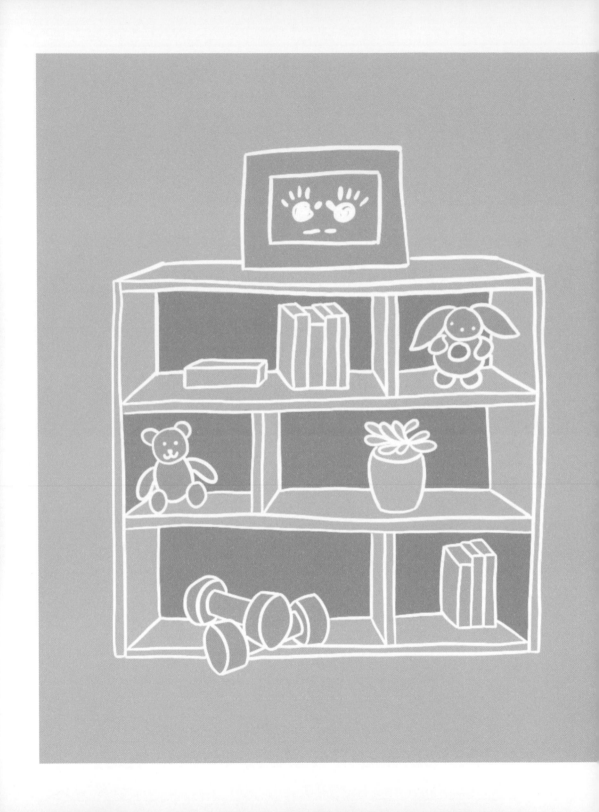

FOURTH TRIMESTER

The early weeks and months

Who even knew there was a fourth trimester?
I certainly didn't before I worked with new and
expectant mums, but it is very real and important. It is
essentially those first 12 or so weeks after the birth,
though there is no end date set in stone.

WHAT TO EXPECT IN
THE FOURTH TRIMESTER

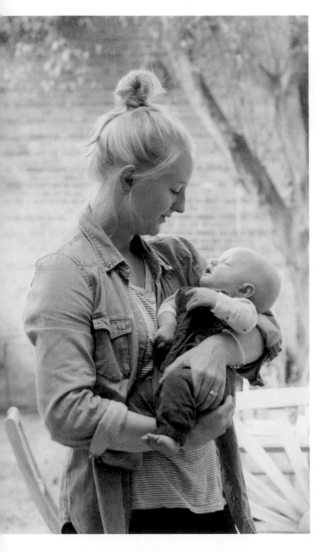

Huge congratulations! You might be reading this whilst feeding your baby for the umpteenth time today, or trying to keep your eyes open after a disrupted night's sleep, but you have made it – you have your baby in your arms and I couldn't be more thrilled for you.

Before reading further, I want you to stop for a moment and acknowledge how amazing you are. Being launched into a whole new chapter of your life overnight is no joke and it's important to realize how far you've come since peeing on that pregnancy test. But the roller-coaster doesn't stop here. Oh no, you're now on a different one and with a teeny-tiny friend depending on you for every little thing. No pressure at all is it?

AFTER THE BIRTH

You probably spent months thinking about what it would feel like to hold your baby and imagining that huge rush of love that would come over you. If this happened for you, then of course that's wonderful, but if it didn't, then don't worry. It is normal to have a mixture of feelings when holding your baby for the first time. You may have felt exhaustion (very likely), overwhelm, anxiety – and it may be taking longer than expected to feel that complete rush of love. Many parents take time to bond with their baby, so be kind to yourself and patient.

I remember feeling unsure of what to say as soon as my baby was put on my chest. I was in total shock when I saw his face, and discovered that he was a boy. I felt a great deal of pressure to say and do the right thing, which of course doesn't exist. I was exhausted and relieved, and we just stared at each other for a while. That was special enough.

ARRIVING HOME

Arriving home with your new baby is a huge moment, so feel free to be over-whelmed. For the whole pregnancy, I imagined us walking through that door for the first time with our baby, and here we were doing just that! I was filled with so many more emotions than I had anticipated. I think it is perfectly normal to sit staring in disbelief at your baby

once you are away from the hospital madness. How is it that a day or so ago you didn't have a baby and now you are responsible for keeping this little thing alive?

It can feel quite terrifying but you're not alone, and you will be fine! The best advice I was given for the first few days was to have no expectations and take each hour as it comes, as things can change so quickly. In fact, the first few days at home sort of blurred into one. All we did was feed, change, and cuddle this little baby – oh and stare at him lots!

MANAGING VISITORS

Everyone is going to want to rush over to see the baby, but you need to decide what is right for you. We staggered visitors and they only stayed for an hour each, which was perfect.

It's a good idea to buy a jumbo box of teabags and a huge multi-pack of biscuits, so that when visitors start coming by you can point them in the right direction – that is your hosting duties over. They're not expecting a slap-up lunch, so don't even attempt to make one. Don't feel like you have to tidy your house – visitors are there to see you and the baby and won't notice anything else. If they do stay longer than you'd like, ask them to help you with some cooking, emptying the dishwasher, or tidying up – that will either give them a rather large hint to leave or give you some help. Either way it's a win win!

YOUR HORMONES

You thought this was the end of the pregnancy hormones but oh no, they just reached a whole new level. Not only will you get a surge of new hormones when your milk comes in if you choose to breastfeed, but you will also be dealing with them on little to no sleep.

Are you crying for absolutely no reason, but unable to stop? It's bizarre, isn't it? Sometimes you can be just looking at your baby and feeling happy, then all of a sudden you start sobbing uncontrollably. My advice? Let those tears flow, and don't try to diagnose it as anything or try to figure out why you're

crying. The baby blues is a very normal occurrence and usually starts a few days after the birth and can last for a few hours or around a week or so. It can leave you feeling very low and tearful, but it won't last for long. Stay in your pyjamas and lie on the sofa all day if

> JUST TO CLARIFY, YOU ARE A SUPERMUM THAT CAN DO ANYTHING, BUT YOU NEED TO RECOVER FIRST!

that's what you want to do – there is absolutely no judgement from anyone. Be reassured that the baby blues will pass, but if they don't, and these feelings last a lot longer, then don't ignore them (see box, opposite).

YOUR RECOVERY

Spending a week on the sofa is what a midwife would ideally like to see, but it is not always possible. It could be that you have other children, or you just feel the need to be up and about. You have, however, just had a baby so now is the perfect time to let people help you. Don't feel you have to be a supermum. Just to clarify, you *are* a supermum that can do anything, but you need to

recover first! Ask your partner, or whoever is helping you, to bring the baby to you, or when you fancy a cuppa, simply ask for one. You can use the "because I gave birth" reason from now until the end of time! Having said that, it doesn't mean you shouldn't move at all; gentle movement helps any swelling go

POSTNATAL **DEPRESSION**

Postnatal depression is very different to having the baby blues, but still fairly common, affecting 1 in 10 women within a year after the birth. It is important to seek help as soon as you notice any of the following signs:

- **A persistent feeling** of sadness and low mood.
- **Loss of interest in** the wider world.
- **Withdrawing contact** from other people.
- **Problems concentrating** or making decisions (aside from the general tiredness of being a new mum).

- **Difficulty bonding** with your baby.
- **Dark thoughts** such as harming yourself or your baby.

The symptoms can take a while to become apparent, but often the GP, midwife, or health visitor will recognize them and refer you for specialist help. If they don't, contact your GP to discuss how you are feeling. Often women are afraid of appearing like a bad or ungrateful mother, but they shouldn't – postnatal depression is a common condition and there is help and support available.

PHYSICAL RECOVERY
AFTER THE BIRTH

This is your time to go slow, lap up your newborn, and give your body the chance it deserves to heal and recover. Whether your birth went to plan or was the opposite of how you had imagined it, your body has been through a lot. So what is going on during this time?

In the initial days your womb returns to its original size prior to pregnancy through contractions, which you may feel

> DURING THE INITIAL DAYS IT IS COMMON TO FEEL A BIT LIKE A RAG DOLL, RATHER FLOPPY WITH LIMITED TUMMY STRENGTH.

more so when breastfeeding, if you choose to do that. As this happens, your other organs, which moved to accommodate your growing baby, slowly return to where they were. During the initial days it is common to feel a bit like a rag doll, rather floppy with limited tummy strength. Your body will also still

be losing blood (known as lochia) and your midwives will keep an eye on this with you.

Most women will have a wound to care for, either in the vaginal tissues and pelvic floor muscles for a vaginal delivery, or in the lower tummy for a Caesarean.

VAGINAL DELIVERY

After a vaginal delivery, you can be left feeling like you want to send an SOS for your perineum and vulva! My top tips to help you are:

- **Sitting:** Roll up two towels and place them on a chair or sofa under your thighs so your perineum isn't in contact with the chair. This takes pressure off any stitches, grazes, or swelling.
- **Ice:** Get a clean sanitary pad, wet it with water, and freeze it. Wrap it in a flannel and hold it over your perineum for 5–10 minutes maximum. Do this every few hours.
- **Pelvic floor exercises:** Gentle contractions (see page 76) can help manage swelling, but also start reconnection and strengthening.

- **Painkillers:** It's normal not to want to take pain relief for too long, but it makes all the difference and keeping on top of pain, rather than chasing pain, is really helpful during this time.
- **Movement:** Move little and often.
- **Doing a poo:** Don't strain to open your bowels. Raise your feet up onto a little stool and lean forwards. This helps your pelvic floor relax and makes it easier for you to do a poo. You can use a clean maternity pad to support stitches, whilst you open your bowels.
- **Doing a wee:** Drink lots of water to keep your urine diluted and have a squirty bottle of water handy to flush the area, this helps to reduce stinging.
- **Cleaning:** Use the showerhead to gently wash the area. Use water only and avoid perfumed soaps. Then dab dry with a towel. Change your maternity pads regularly as well.

Don't underestimate the discomfort of 'just grazes'. Six weeks can feel like forever while your body is healing. If your recovery takes longer, don't worry – everyone is different. If you have any severe pain that isn't eased by regular painkillers, or you notice a bad smell from your vagina, seek immediate medical attention; it can indicate an infection.

CAESAREAN

It is important to take extra care after a Caesarean. My top tips to help you are:
- **Early mobilization:** If you have your baby in the morning, try to get up that afternoon for a short walk or to sit in a chair, with guidance from your medical team. Getting out of bed is helpful for managing swelling and therefore pain.
- **Bed transfers:** To get out of bed, roll on to your side and push up with your arms like you would have done towards the end of pregnancy.
- **Scar support:** If you need to cough, sneeze, or laugh, have a blanket or towel at the ready over your scar and apply pressure to support the wound.
- **Sleeping:** Pop a pillow under your knees if you are lying on your back, or under your tummy if you are lying on your side, to prevent any pulling or dragging on the scar in the early days.

TAKING TIME **TO HEAL**

If you're used to exercising, not being able to return to it straight away may make you panic. However, I'd encourage you to stay mindful of the ongoing changes your body is going through. On top of that, you have hormonal changes, especially whilst breastfeeding, and sleep deprivation, which is not to be underestimated.

I often say to new mums, "If you were to tear your hamstring, how would you approach your return to exercise? I am sure you would see a physiotherapist and ask them to help guide you back to exercise safely. You wouldn't go for a run after six weeks." Your pelvic floor and tummy need the same approach after having a baby, so try to view your fourth healing and rehabilitation trimester in this way.

Soft tissue healing takes around six weeks after the birth, which is why the recommendation is to wait around this amount of time before returning to more formal workouts and exercise. However, be aware that healing can be delayed if you have experienced any infections.

Equally it is understood from research that the healing process after a Caesarean, including the uterine scar, will continue beyond six weeks so that is why we don't rush back to our pre-baby workouts straight away.

It is not just the scars we need to think about, but the changes to the muscles of the tummy and pelvic floor and the connective tissue, called fascia. They have all changed in length and strength, and do not return to their pre-baby state at six weeks.

Expert guidelines recommend that returning to running and impact exercise is not advisable before three months postpartum and to monitor for any symptoms of pelvic floor dysfunction (see box on page 203) on return.

SIX WEEKS CAN FEEL LIKE FOREVER WHILE YOUR BODY IS HEALING. IF YOUR RECOVERY TAKES LONGER, DON'T WORRY – EVERYONE IS DIFFERENT.

- **Doing a poo:** Trapped wind can be more painful than the scar, so movement can help. Don't put it off when you have the urge to do a poo.
- **Pain relief:** Keep taking the pain relief for as long as you need – you may need to do so for a few weeks.
- **Lifting:** The advice is to aim not to lift anything heavier than your baby for around six weeks , which isn't easy if you have older children, or have to handle car seats, but it's a helpful guide.
- **Pelvic floor exercises:** Start these (see page 202) once the catheter is out and you have done your first wee.
- **Help:** Accept all the help you can get, especially if you have children already. Plan childcare in advance if you can.

- **Driving:** Check with your insurance company, but usually you can start driving from 4–6 weeks after the birth. You need to be able to do an emergency stop and wear the seatbelt comfortably.
- **Movement:** Pottering around the house is often enough movement, but you can venture out for a short walk. Slow and steady wins the race. Remember that painkillers and anti-inflammatories can mask symptoms.

SCAR MASSAGE

Scar massage isn't often talked about, but can really help a number of symptoms. If you have any concerns about doing this or need some individualized advice, consult a pelvic health physiotherapist (see page 203).

Vaginal scar massage

Like any other scars, vaginal scars can become tight and uncomfortable as they heal and can be made worse by the sensitivity of the vaginal tissues. Only do vaginal scar massages after six weeks and once the wound has fully healed. Use the same technique as perineal massage (see page 154), but focus on any sensitive or tight areas.

Doing vaginal scar massage is beneficial in several ways:

- **Sensation:** Scars in the vaginal area can be highly sensitive and sore once they heal; gentle massage can help to desensitize them. This is particularly helpful if sex has been sore or uncomfortable since birth.
- **Reduce muscle restriction**: Second-, third-, and fourth-degree tears involve the pelvic floor muscles. Scars within muscles can restrict their movement; therefore improving mobility of the scar and surrounding connective tissue helps muscle function. Sometimes women struggle to improve their pelvic floor strength as the muscles are restricted by their scars – after some scar and muscle release, pelvic floor movement and symptoms improve.
- **Improve sex:** Due to sensitivity and tightness, vaginal scars can be tender and therefore make sex uncomfortable. Massage can help with this.

- **Reconnect with your body:** Vaginal scar massage can help you to reconnect with your body postnatally, but I am aware that not all women may be comfortable with this.

Sometimes scars overheal, producing granulation tissue – this is usually bright red and tender to the touch. If the area feels raw when you touch, massage, or have sex, seek medical advice.

Caesarean scar massage

It can be difficult to imagine touching your scar in the early days and weeks after a Caesarean, especially if you had an emergency one or a traumatic experience. There is no pressure to start massage, but sometimes women find it helpful once they begin.

After six weeks, start with gentle circles around the lower tummy using a natural oil. You can work just above the scar, not directly on it, if you prefer. Then, as you feel more confident, move on to the scar and using two fingers together sweep side to side approximately 10 times, then make little circles round and round along the whole length of the scar 10 times, and then up and down along the length of the scar 10 times.

As the weeks go by and you feel comfortable and more confident, work up to gently pulling the scar from above and below, and then try picking it up between your fingers and rolling it. As you are doing this massage, you may feel some areas are tighter, so focus on these.

You can massage over your clothes, rather that directly on the skin, if this feels more comfortable for you physically and emotionally.

Caesarean scar massage can be beneficial in a number of ways, including:

- **Sensation and numbness:** Nerves are damaged during surgery, leaving numbness. Touching the skin and scar, including using different textures, can help sensation to return.
- **Manage swelling:** Sometimes you can find there is a pocket of swelling above the scar. Gently massaging this area can help.
- **Reduce muscle restriction:** Scars restrict connective tissue, which can then restrict surrounding muscles.

Improving mobility of the scar and surrounding connective tissue helps muscle function, including diastasis (see pages 113 and 206).

- **Reduce tugging:** It is normal to feel tugging and tightness in the scar and massage can reduce this.
- **Help overhang:** When a scar is tight, it can increase the look of overhang on your abdomen. Massage can help to reduce this.

FLASHBACKS

Sometimes touching a scar, whether it is a vaginal scar or abdominal one, can bring up emotions or for some trigger memories or flashbacks, especially if you had a traumatic birth. If this happens, please do speak to someone. You can access support via your GP or health visitor, so please don't suffer alone.

NAVIGATING YOUR
CHANGED BODY

Were you shocked to be left with a bump after the birth? Or breasts that were twice the size? There is no knowing how your body is going to look after having a baby, but try not to fixate on it too much in those early weeks. Your body needs time to recover; things will have moved around and need time to find their way back to their original place.

> YOUR BODY WON'T 'SNAP BACK' IMMEDIATELY AND WHY SHOULD IT? IT HAS JUST GROWN A HUMAN BEING!

There is a lot of hype in the media about who has 'snapped back' after birth and, to be honest, I hate the fascination with it. Of course your body won't 'snap back' immediately and why should it? Look at what it has been through – it has grown a human being!

There is no such thing as snapping back, even if it looks like it from the outside. Think how far your uterus had to stretch. It is completely unrealistic to expect it all to return to how it was within a few days or weeks, so let's nip that in the bud right now. No comparing ourselves to celebrities, okay?

MAKING ADJUSTMENTS

I am not saying you have to love your postpartum body – that is also totally unrealistic. We don't all love our bodies every single day normally, so why should we now. I am just encouraging you to be patient and kind to yourself.

It's perfectly okay not to like the look of your tummy right now and wish your body was firmer. I certainly found it strange to all of a sudden have a squidgy tummy after months of just about getting used to a tight bump. Not only am I now navigating motherhood, which is a rollercoaster in itself, but I am also doing it in a body that I don't really recognize either. Of course it can feel tough.

It really helped me to find some clothes that didn't grip too tightly – I have found maxi dresses, baggy tops, and sweatshirts a godsend in these early months. There is no point trying to squeeze into clothes that aren't going to fit you just yet.

Maybe treat yourself to a nice new outfit or two that make you feel fabulous, even when you have had no sleep. Online shopping at 3am can be a great way to stay awake while you're feeding. The bonus is you'll probably forget that you've ordered anything, so when it arrives it is like a gift you didn't know was coming. I speak from experience here!

BEWARE SOCIAL MEDIA

Social media is a wonderful tool for navigating pregnancy and motherhood. I really believe that the community of mums you can find there is huge and so supportive. Not so helpful are the posts of celebrities leaving hospital in their jeans after giving birth, or being photographed in a bikini in the first couple of weeks.

Remember that everyone is different – we all have different genetics – and be aware of the photoshopping and carefully planned photo angles often used to show these new mums in their best light. I tell the new mothers I work with to do a big social media cull and only follow accounts that inspire them of people they can relate to right now. You can come back to follow some of the other accounts at a later date, but there is no point scrolling through countless feeds that make you feel worse when you may already be a little vulnerable.

You have control over what you see when you scroll, so make sure that every time you turn on your phone you enjoy what comes up and aren't left feeling inadequate. I felt so liberated after I did a social media cull and would thoroughly recommend it – be ruthless!

I'd encourage you to keep this in mind in the coming months, too. Whether it is how you dress your baby, feed your baby, or how well your baby sleeps, there is always going to be someone doing it differently. It is not always easy, but try to be confident in your decisions and trust your gut. No one knows you or your baby better, not even someone you've never met on Instagram!

EXERCISE IN THE
FOURTH TRIMESTER

Many new mums ask when they can start exercising again and the answer is "It depends"– on how your body recovers from pregnancy and the type of exercise. I always recommend six weeks is the absolute minimum amount of time you need off exercise, but it could be longer if you don't feel ready.

> IF YOU ARE FEELING GREAT AND RARING TO GO, THEN IT IS JUST ABOUT STARTING BACK WITH THE RIGHT KIND OF EXERCISE.

Don't feel that on the morning of the six-week mark you are all 'fixed' and ready to go – ease yourself in. I found six weeks came round surprisingly quickly. I was not raring to exercise like I thought I would be. I was exhausted and, if I'm honest, a little apprehensive. I had been building up my walks and enjoying those. At six weeks I did some gentle movement and was surprised at how much my muscles ached for the next few days; this served as a reminder to take it easy.

If you are feeling great and raring to go, then it is just about starting back with the right kind of exercise. Don't go out for a run on your first day back; your body will not thank you for it. You could begin with the exercises in this chapter and then do some bodyweight work just to build up your strength again. You could repeat the workouts earlier in this book to get you going, but take it at a pace that feels good for you and listen to your body.

The UK's Chief Medical Officer advises to build up to 150 minutes of moderate intensity activity each week after having a baby, slowly introducing muscle strengthening twice a week. Don't underestimate how active you will be and are as a mother; so remember every activity counts, not just 'workouts'.

BREASTFEEDING

It is natural to question whether exercise impacts breastfeeding, as there can be conflicting advice in this area. Be reassured that it is absolutely safe to exercise while you are breastfeeding; it does not impact your milk supply or the minerals and nutrients in the milk. It is, however, important that you keep yourself well hydrated and eat nutritious food. When you are breastfeeding, you need to keep well hydrated anyway, so if you are exercising and sweating, then you just have to keep topped up.

There is some evidence that with maximum effort exercise, lactic acid levels are higher for up to 90 minutes afterwards and this can make the milk taste slightly different, but this won't harm your baby. You are likely to be working at a more moderate intensity level for a while anyway, in which case this would not even occur.

If you are doing high-impact exercise, like running or jumping, ensure you have a supportive sports bra and aim to feed before you start, for your own comfort.

WALKING

I have always thought that going for a walk was the easiest and most gentle thing you could do, but in the fourth trimester it can feel like quite a challenge. Aside from the fact that you need to time

POSTNATAL **CHECK-UP**

A lot of GP practices offer a 6–8 week postnatal check-up, but this is not standard practice for all areas of the UK. The following may be discussed:

- **Mental health:** This includes any birth trauma or feeding issues and any signs of postnatal depression (see page 191) that you may be experiencing.
- **Physical health:** Checking your vaginal bleeding has stopped or if you have any concerns regarding your wounds. These may not be routinely checked, so bring them to your GP's attention if you are worried. This is also the time to raise any concerns about incontinence or prolapse if you have these.
- **Contraception:** Resuming sex may be the last thing on your mind, but it is important to discuss contraception at your postnatal check.

it in-between feeds and nappy changes, for the first couple of weeks a short, slow walk can be exhausting. Be realistic about distances because if you head out too far, you may feel too tired to get back. It's better to set yourself time goals – maybe 10 minutes one day, then 15 minutes the next, and so on. That way you can check how your body feels as

> YOU MIGHT EVEN BE ABLE TO GRAB A COFFEE AND LISTEN TO A PODCAST OR MEET A FRIEND – IMAGINE THAT? JUST LIKE OLD TIMES!

you go. If possible, go with someone the first couple of times, in case you come over dizzy or need help with the baby.

Once you get past those first few walks and build up a little more strength to go further, you will realize that walking is a brilliant way to be active. Firstly, your baby will hopefully love sleeping in the buggy, and secondly this is your time for some peace and quiet. Getting fresh air and some time to yourself can do wonders for your mood – you might even be able to grab a coffee and listen to a podcast or meet a friend. Imagine that? Just like old times! But seriously, I have always been a fan of walking, and I'm even more so now. Every day I try to get out for a walk and it never fails to lift my mood or make me feel more awake after a rough night with not much sleep.

PELVIC FLOOR EXERCISES

The midwife will encourage you to do a wee within the first six hours and you can resume pelvic floor exercises after that. You may be concerned if you have stitches, but gentle pelvic floor contractions can, in fact, help with swelling, pain, and healing. If you've had a Caesarean, there may be some lower abdominal discomfort, so go steady.

It is also really normal not to feel much in the early days, but keep trying. Don't go pumping out 100 pelvic floor

RED **FLAGS**

When returning to movement, activity, and exercise after having a baby, it is important to look out for the following:

- Vaginal bleeding restarting
- Incontinence of urine or faeces
- Heaviness or dragging sensation within the vagina
- Ongoing or new pelvic girdle or back pain

If you experience any of these, or other symptoms that are new, then please do speak to a GP or physiotherapist.

SPECIALIST **HELP**

Seeing a pelvic health physiotherapist during the fourth trimester is beneficial, although as this is not available for all on the NHS I am aware it comes with a financial commitment.

If you are symptomatic of pelvic floor dysfunction (see the symptoms listed above), then you can access this support via your GP. Referral may not always be possible but the National Institute for Clinical Excellence (NICE) guidelines state that pelvic floor physiotherapy should be first-line treatment for incontinence or prolapse, so it should definitely be considered.

If you do not have symptoms, a postnatal check is still advised; it is the only true way to understand exactly how your body is recovering and how best to return to the exercise you love. The best way to find a private physiotherapist is via the Squeezy App Directory Online (www.squeezyapp.com) or the Mummy MOT website (www.themummymot.com).

It is important to know that if you have symptoms of pelvic floor dysfunction, it does not mean that exercise, especially impact exercise, is off the table forever. You just need the right support and advice to guide you back. Running and impact is not bad for your pelvic floor, but it needs to be able to meet the demands of these movements.

exercises on day one, as slow and steady definitely wins the race. It can be tempting in the postnatal period when everything feels a bit different, or you have some incontinence, to get into a pattern of holding the pelvic floor muscles, but remember the let-go is as important as the squeeze.

Gradually work up to doing your short and long contractions (see pages 76–77), aiming for 10 of each type three times a day. The best time is when you are feeding the baby as it is a good prompt and you will be sitting down. If, however, you are struggling to feel any contraction, try lying on your side.

In the coming weeks, work up to doing the exercises while standing, as this is an important part of your pelvic floor rehabilitation.

If you experience any symptoms of pelvic floor dysfunction during your return to exercise – usually this would present as urinary or faecal incontinence, or a prolapse, which can feel like a heaviness or dragging sensation within the vagina – please do not accept it as normal or part of the postpartum period.

SEEING YOUR ABS MIGHT FEEL LIKE A DISTANT MEMORY BUT, JUST AS IT WAS IN THE PREGNANCY, THE CORE IS VERY MUCH STILL THERE AND DOING AN IMPORTANT JOB.

Speak to your GP to discuss referral to a pelvic health physiotherapist (see page 203) or seek one out privately. You really don't need to suffer in silence and there is so much help out there. We know from research that there is a significant link between pelvic floor dysfunction and depression, and it is therefore essential we address these symptoms for our physical and mental wellbeing.

RE-ENGAGING THE CORE

Seeing your abs might feel like a distant memory but, just as it was in the pregnancy, the core is very much still there and doing an important job. You can start to gently wake it up a little bit again in the first few weeks after the birth. We are not talking doing crunches or going to the gym – just using your breath to reconnect to those deep core muscles.

Everyday activities such as getting out of bed should still be done carefully – turning on to your side. Keep up those good habits that you learned in pregnancy as they will do wonders for helping your body to recover.

Start with breathing

Now I know this sounds super-dull and not really where you want to start, but effective breathing is key to rebuilding core strength and will really help in the months and years to come.

As we exhale, there is a natural activation of the pelvic floor and transversus adbominis (see page 206), so by simply doing diaphragmatic breathing during this time you are helping your muscles to rehabilitate. Amazing right?

Sit or lie down, and try not to fall asleep (I realize this is easier said than done in the fourth trimester!) Start by placing one hand on your upper chest

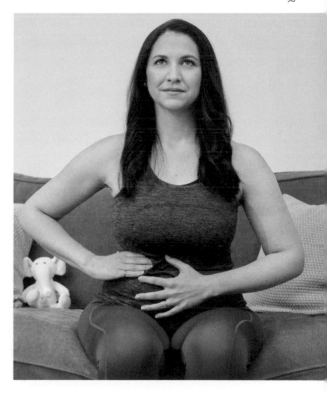

and one hand on your tummy, and take a breath in. Where do you feel most movement? When we are stressed, we tend to breathe into our upper chest. We want to try to send that breath down into the tummy. So now pop one hand on the side of your ribs and keep one

USING THE BREATH
WITHIN EXERCISE AND
MOVEMENT IS SO
POWERFUL, ESPECIALLY
POSTNATALLY.

hand on your tummy. Take a slow deep breath in now, widening the ribs into your hands and letting your tummy expand.

You can do this breathing exercise at any point in your day, it really helps to calm you after a tiring day and night.

Building a core connection

Using the breath within exercise and movement is so powerful, especially postnatally, so now we are going to introduce the breath with your pelvic floor and transversus abdominis (deep abdominals) connection.

The pelvic floor is activated by thinking about holding wind, and doing this on an exhale breath can help activation. For the transversus abdominis everyone will find different cues helpful, but the cue that many of the women

I work with find useful is to imagine two magnets on the front of your pelvic bones. You are gently drawing them together as you exhale. If you take two fingers just in and a few centimetres down from the front of your pelvis, you can often feel the muscle tighten under your finger.

This is the foundation of all the other exercises that are in this chapter (see pages 210–215), so practise it whenever you get a moment. You don't have to lie down, but you might find it the easiest position to begin with.

Diastasis

Diastasis rectus abdominis is the scientific term given to the stretching or separation that occurs between the rectus abdominus, your six-pack muscles, during pregnancy (see pages 113–114) and it isn't something to be feared. In fact, we should embrace it and celebrate how our body has adapted to grow our baby!

Around one-third of women will need support and rehabilitation for diastasis after birth, with the other two-thirds having natural improvement, so for most women it isn't an issue. However, it is worth being aware of it and doing the step-by-step check outlined below.

Always keep in mind the key message, though – it is not just about how far apart the muscles sit, but actually the tension of the connective tissue between them.

When you return to exercise, especially exercise you may label 'core' exercises, keep an eye out for any doming (see page 114) or any of the tissues between the tummy muscles dropping down into the tummy. You may not always get doming upwards like you might have seen while you were pregnant.

How to check yourself:

1. Lie on your back on the floor, with your knees bent.

2. Gently lift your head and at the same time use one hand to feel down the centre of your tummy, from the bottom of your breast bone, all the way down to your pubic bone. It is important to check the whole way along the linea alba (connective tissue between the muscles) as it is possible to have different areas of separation.

3. You are feeling for how many fingers you can fit between the six-pack muscles, as well as how far you can drop them down between the muscles. Look for tension in the connective tissue, as well as how far apart the muscles are.

4. If you feel you can drop down quite far, try doing a contraction of your pelvic floor and see if that improves the tension you can feel under your fingers. If that doesn't change anything, try the TVA (transversus abdominis) engagement (see opposite) to see if that improves the tension under your fingers.

5. If when checking yourself you feel that you are able to drop down between the muscles, you don't feel much tension there, and cannot change this by doing your pelvic floor contraction or deep abdominal activation as described here, then seek an assessment with a physiotherapist, either via your GP or privately (see box on page 203).

FOURTH TRIMESTER
EXERCISES

The postnatal exercises in this section can be done in the comfort of your own home, perhaps when your baby is napping or when someone is on hand to help. Time is very precious with a newborn, so don't feel that you need to set aside a big chunk of time – little and often is what you're aiming for. After the six-week mark, there is no right time to start doing postnatal exercises – see how your body feels as you recover and when you decide the time is right, give them a go. Once you have tried each one and are starting to feel more confident, you might like to create a mini sequence that you can do when you have more time. Try 10 repetitions of each exercise and see how you get on, but if that feels too much right now, do as many as feels right for you. Always listen to your body.

POSTNATAL
EXERCISES

These are gentle but very effective exercises, and the bonus is you will get to lie down on the mat. Stay focused, though, so that you don't fall asleep!

THREAD
THE NEEDLE

This works on the movement in your upper back, which might feel stiff from feeding and carrying your baby.

Come on to your hands and knees in a four-point kneeling position (see overleaf).

Reach one arm through the gap between your other arm and leg (this is the eye of the needle – your free arm is the thread).

Reach through as far as you can, while keeping your hips still.

Then reach your arm up towards the ceiling.

Repeat on the other side.

AT YOUR
OWN PACE

Only do postnatal exercises when you feel ready to do so, and not before six weeks after the birth.

BENT KNEE **FALLOUTS**

This introduces some gentle challenge and is a lovely way to start working on pelvic floor and deep abdominal activation with movement.

Lie on your back and rock your pelvis forwards and backwards to find the mid-point between the two extremes of movement.

Inhale to prepare.

Exhale, allowing one knee to gently fall out to the side. With this exhale and movement, engage your pelvic floor and deep abdominals gently.

Only take the knee as far as you can control it without letting your pelvis rock from side to side.

The leg that is not moving should remain still.

Bring the leg back into the middle and repeat on the other side.

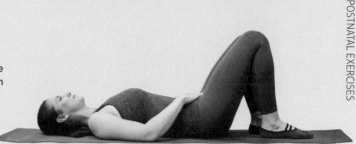

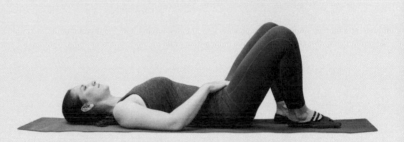

BRIDGING **EXERCISE**

This strengthens your bottom muscles as you push up.

Lie on your back with your knees bent.

Inhale to prepare, then as you exhale push through your heels. Engage your pelvic floor and deep abdominals gently as you do this.

Don't push too high and keep a straight line from your knees to your neck.

Slowly lower to the mat and let your tummy and pelvic floor relax before repeating.

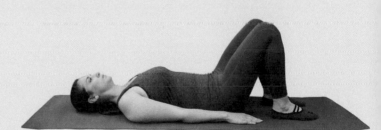

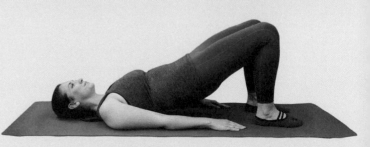

POSTNATAL
EXERCISES

You will find yourself on the floor a lot with your baby, now and in the coming months, so you can try a few of these exercises when you are!

4-POINT
ARM RAISES

This works your tummy muscles as well as the muscles around your shoulders.

Come on to your hands and knees in a four-point kneeling position. Your hips should be above your knees and your shoulders above your wrists.

Lift one arm up as your exhale, engaging your pelvic floor and deep abdominals.

Don't let your body rock from side to side and keep your neck long, so your head doesn't drop down towards the mat.

Relax as you bring your hands back down to the mat.

Repeat on the other side.

AT YOUR
OWN PACE

Only do postnatal exercises when you feel ready to do so, and not before six weeks after the birth.

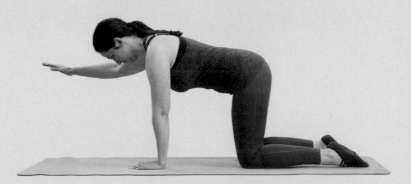

LEG **SLIDES**

This can look and seem like a simple exercise, but you will definitely feel your muscles working.

Lie on your back with your knees bent.

Inhale to prepare.

Exhale as you straighten one leg and engage your pelvic floor and deep abdominals.

Straighten your leg as far as you can before your lower back starts to lift off the mat.

Inhale as you bring your leg back to the starting position and let your pelvic floor and tummy relax.

Repeat on the other side.

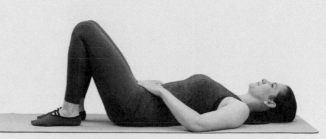

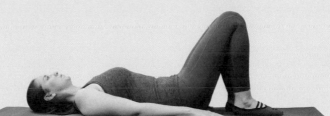

HEAD **LIFT**

This helps to strengthen your tummy muscles and train for movements like getting out of bed without rolling, as you will have done at the end of pregnancy.

Lie on your back with your knees bent.

Engage your pelvic floor and deep abdominals as you exhale and gently lift your head up, bringing your chin towards your chest.

Hold the lifted position for a moment, then relax back down.

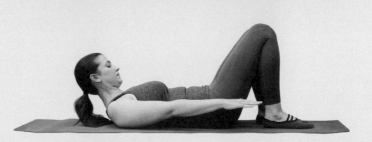

POSTNATAL EXERCISES

Bending and lifting will make up a good part of your day now that you are caring for a baby. These exercises help you to train for this and strengthen your body.

SIT TO **STAND**

This is a great exercise that you should feel working your bottom muscles as well as your legs.

Sit on the edge of a chair with your feet just behind your knees.

Lean your whole body forwards from your hips.

Keep your back straight and push up through your heels into standing as you exhale.

Gently return to a sitting position and repeat the exercise.

AT YOUR OWN PACE

Only do postnatal exercises when you feel ready to do so, and not before six weeks after the birth.

SPLIT STANCE
SQUAT

This is a movement you will do a lot as you care for your baby, so it is great to use it as an exercise as well.

Step into a split squat position as shown.

Inhale as you bend your legs and lower down.

Exhale as you push up into standing.

Repeat on the other side.

DEADLIFT
EXERCISE

You will find yourself doing a deadlift movement regularly when picking up car seats, and tidying up toys and washing off the floor.

Start in a relaxed standing position.

Lean forwards into the deadlift position as shown. There will be a slight bend of the knees.

Exhale as you come into standing and squeeze your bottom muscles.

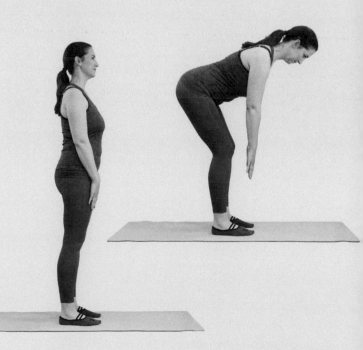

GOOD LUCK

I hope you will dip in and out of this book as you need it, but here is a reminder of some of the key points for easy reference.

1. Listen to your body... it will tell you when something isn't right. Tune in to it and respond by resting or seeking specialist advice.

2. Try not to compare... your bump, your symptoms, your cravings, your postpartum body. We are all different.

3. It's ok not to love being pregnant every day... it doesn't mean you are not grateful – some days are harder than others and you are allowed to get frustrated and 'hormotional' about it.

4. Trust your instincts... You really do know yourself and your baby best.

5. It is ok to cry A LOT... and find the transition to motherhood hard. You cannot possibly enjoy every minute, as some people love to advise, but just take each day as it comes. It is a rollercoaster, but you will look back and think, wow, it was worth it.

We can never be fully prepared for pregnancy and motherhood – there are many surprises along the way, but I found

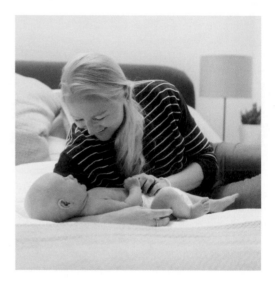

it comforting and reassuring to know that other people were on this rollercoaster with me. Through my own pregnancy and by working with so many wonderful expectant mums, I am constantly reminded that a woman's body is incredible and I have a whole new level of respect for it. I hope you do too. Growing a baby is no easy job and pregnancy can feel seriously overwhelming at times, so it has been my pleasure to go through it with you. Good luck to you, wherever you are on your pregnancy and motherhood journey.

RESOURCES

Apps
Freya App
Timing contractions and hypnobirthing

NHS Squeezy App
Pelvic floor exercise reminders

Pregnancy+
Daily pregnancy tracker

Books
Expecting Better by Emily Oster
(Orion, 2018)

Happy Mum, Happy Baby by Giovanna
Fletcher (Coronet, 2018)

Mind Over Mother by Anna Mathur
(Piatkus, 2020)

Pregnancy After Loss by Zoe Clarke-
Coates (Orion, 2020)

The Positive Birth Book by Milli Hill
(Pinter & Martin Ltd, 2017)

The Supermum Myth by Anya Hayes
(White Ladder Press, 2017)

*Your Baby, Your Birth: Hypnobirthing
Skills for Every Birth* by Hollie de Cruz
(Vermilion, 2018)

Websites
Mummy MOT
www.themummymot.com
(specialist postnatal examination)

Squeezy App Directory
www.squeezyapp.com
(how to find a physiotherapist near you)

The Pelvic Obstetric Gynaecological
Physiotherapists (POGP)
www.thepogp.co.uk
(free information leaflets)

INDEX

DEDICATION

I've always dreamed of being a mum, and I count myself extremely lucky that I now am one. This book is for everyone who supported me through the many ups and downs in the journey to get here. It would have been a very different story without you.

ACKNOWLEDGEMENTS

This book would not have been possible without my wonderful husband George who has supported me in sharing our miscarriage and pregnancy story, in the hope that it might help others. Thank you for not only supporting me through our own pregnancy, but for encouraging me to pursue my dream of writing this book, and I am delighted to be now navigating the ups and downs of parenthood with you.

A huge thank you to Clare for getting so passionately involved with this book. You are a dream to work with, so full of knowledge, and I'm so grateful you shared my vision for this project.

Thank you to my gorgeous models Emily and Zeri, who posed for hundreds of exercises, in a heat wave, without a single complaint. You looked radiant and strong, and I am so happy to have your bumps in this book alongside mine.

To all the women I have worked with for the past 10 years, thank you for showing me your incredible strength and resilience that inspires me to keep going even when things are tough.

To my family and friends, every single one of you, thank you for the never-ending love and support you have given me with this book and all the other mad ideas I come up with.

I am so glad that Lauren approached me and encouraged me to write this book – thank you for giving me the confidence to pursue it.

I am unbelievably grateful for the amazing team at DK who have been so patient with me – taking on a pregnant, first-time author and working with me on editing through the newborn days was a risk, but I am thrilled that you took it. Thank you... Steph for believing in my idea and helping me bring it to life; the design team Karen, Max, and Bess for making the book look as beautiful as it does; Claire for the wonderful photography; Amy for the illustrations; Dawn for editing – you are one patient lady, receiving my edits during the night feeds and working with me around baby naps, or lack thereof, thank you for being a joy to work with. There are so many more amazing people behind the scenes, so thank you to you all!

And finally... Thank you to Alfie for hanging on in there and making me the mum I am today. You make me happier than I ever imagined I could be.

Charlie Barker

Founder & Managing Director
Bumps & Burpees
www.bumpsandburpees.com
@bumpsandburpees